ATLAS OF
BREAST IMAGING

ATLAS OF BREAST IMAGING

Daniel B. Kopans, M.D.
Director of Breast Imaging
Department of Radiology
Massachusetts General Hospital
Associate Professor of Radiology
Harvard Medical School
Boston, Massachusetts

LIPPINCOTT WILLIAMS & WILKINS
A **Wolters Kluwer** Company

Philadelphia · Baltimore · New York · London
Buenos Aires · Hong Kong · Sydney · Tokyo

Acquisitions Editor: James D. Ryan
Developmental Editor: Mary Beth Murphy
Manufacturing Manager: Tim Reynolds
Production Manager: Jodi Borgenicht
Production Editor: Deirdre Marino-Vasquez
Cover Designer: Sandy Mohindru
Indexer: Susan Thomas
Compositor: Maryland Composition
Printed: Quebecor Kingsport

Printed and bound in the United States

9 8 7 6 5 4 3 2 1

Library of Congress Cataloging-in-Publication Data

Kopans, Daniel B.
    Atlas of breast imaging / Daniel B. Kopans.
        p. cm.
    Includes index.
    Complement to: Breast imaging / Daniel B. Kopans. 2nd ed. ©1998.
    ISBN 0-7817-1720-5 (hardcover)
    1. Breast—Imaging. 2. Breast—Cancer—Diagnosis. 3. Breast—Cancer—
Imaging—Atlases. 4. Breast—Imaging—Atlases. 5. Breast—Radiography—Atlases.
  6. Diagnostic imaging—Atlases. I. Kopans, Daniel B. Breast imaging. II. Title.
    [DNLM: 1. Breast Neoplasms—diagnosis atlases. 2. Diagnostic Imaging atlases.
  3. Mammography—methods atlases. WP 17 K83a 1998]
    RC280.B8K67   1997 Suppl.
    616.99′4490754—dc21
    DNLM/DLC
    for Library of Congress   98-43303
                                             CIP

Care has been taken to confirm the accuracy of the information presented and to describe generally accepted practices. However, the author and publisher are not responsible for errors or omissions or for any consequences from application of the information in this book and make no warranty, expressed or implied, with respect to the contents of the publication.

The author and publisher have exerted every effort to ensure that drug selection and dosage set forth in this text are in accordance with current recommendations and practice at the time of publication. However, in view of ongoing research, changes in government regulations, and the constant flow of information relating to drug therapy and drug reactions, the reader is urged to check the package insert for each drug for any change in indications and dosage and for added warnings and precautions. This is particularly important when the recommended agent is a new or infrequently employed drug.

Some drugs and medical devices presented in this publication have Food and Drug Administration (FDA) clearance for limited use in restricted research settings. It is the responsibility of the health care provider to ascertain the FDA status of each drug or device planned for use in their clinical practice.

Contents

Preface

The ability to detect and diagnose breast cancer is a function of learning and experience. Radiologists are, for the most part, visually oriented. My textbook *Breast Imaging, Second Edition*, published by Lippincott-Raven, Philadelphia, in 1998 was written to provide an in-depth discussion of the many issues and details involved in detection and diagnosis. This *Atlas of Breast Imaging* has been provided to complement the cases described in *Breast Imaging*. Whenever possible these cases provide either histological confirmation, or long term (over two years) follow-up, of the lesions.

The sections are organized along the categories defined in the American College of Radiology Breast Imaging Reporting and Data System (BIRADS), and represent my interpretation of the BIRADS Lexicon. BIRADS is designed to be flexible and improved with time. The reader is referred to the BIRADS document for the ACR definitions, official language, and descriptions to be used. A discussion of BIRADS can be found in *Breast Imaging, Second Edition* (pp. 762–790).

The organization of this atlas is based on BIRADS. The main sections provide examples of the various mammographic and ultrasonographic findings that might be encountered in a busy clinical practice. Teaching points are provided where appropriate. These are the most valuable parts of the atlas, having been designed to provide the reader with the tools to approach other similar situations.

The atlas opens with a series of screening cases. Screening and the earlier detection of breast cancer is the primary reason for imaging the breast. The cases have been chosen to illustrate a number of the situations encountered in screening. Naturally, it would be impossible to provide examples of all of the possibilities. The lesions found at screening lead to the need to interpret the findings. It is hoped that the atlas will provide information to aid the radiologist who encounters similar situations. BIRADS assessment codes are used as follows:

0. The study is incomplete and additional imaging evaluation is needed.
1. The mammogram is negative.
2. There is a benign finding. The mammogram is negative.
3. There is a finding that is probably benign, but short interval follow-up is suggested. (We use a follow-up schedule of every 6 months for a 2-year period. If the lesion has remained stable over 2 years then it is suggested that the patient return to annual screening.)

4. There is an abnormality that is suspicious, and cytologic or histologic analysis should be considered.
5. There is a lesion that has a high probability of malignancy.

The reader is referred to *Breast Imaging, Second Edition* (pp. 55–100) for an in-depth discussion of the various findings and the details involved in screening and diagnosis.

Since there can be overlapping appearances, these illustrations are meant as references and not as an absolute determinants of histology. The sections are organized along specific characteristics of lesions to facilitate use by the reader.

Section I:
Mammography Screening

The primary role of mammography is to detect cancers earlier among asymptomatic women who have no signs or symptoms of these malignancies. Since breast cancer is relatively uncommon, the radiologist can expect to find only two to ten cancers per 1,000 screening examinations, depending on the age and risk factors of the women being screened and whether this is their first (prevalence) screen or they have been regularly screened before (incidence screen). In addition to breast cancer, approximately 5% to 10% of women will have a benign finding, or a finding that requires additional evaluation before a final assessment can be reached. The cases described in the figures in this section are all asymptomatic women who provide a mix of the kind of findings that can appear on screening mammograms.

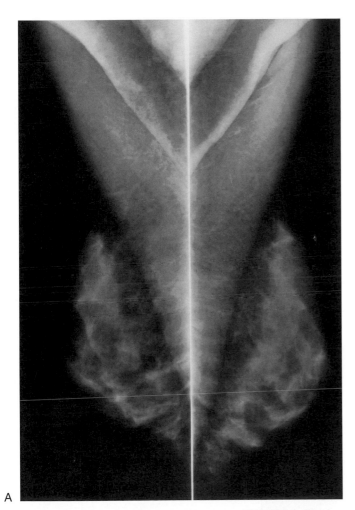 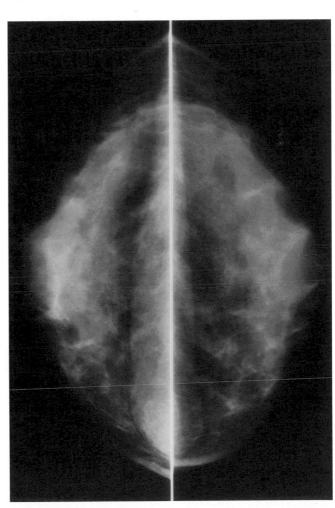

A   B

SC-1. Normal screening mammogram. BIRADS 1. The breasts are well positioned on the MLO (mediolateral oblique) *(A)* and CC (craniocaudal) *(B)* projections. The tissues are well penetrated and symmetrical. No abnormality is seen.

Teaching Point: Most screening mammograms are negative.

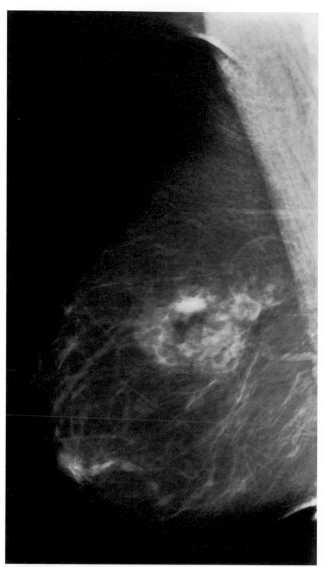

A

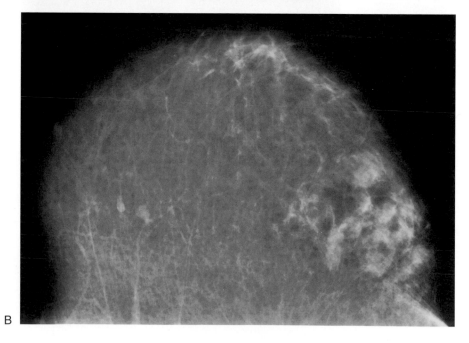

B

SC-2. Superimposed breast tissue (summation shadow). The high-density finding on the MLO *(A)* is probably a benign superimposition of breast tissue since there is no corresponding mass on the CC *(B)* projection. Recall for additional evaluation, however, would be reasonable. This makes this screening study incomplete (BIRADS 0). Additional evaluation proved that the density was, in fact, due to superimposing tissues. No mass was present.

Teaching Points: 1. Superimposed breast tissue is likely when a lesion is seen only in one projection, assuming the images are properly positioned and exposed. 2. If a lesion is seen on the CC projection and not on the MLO, it is more likely to be real than if it is seen on the MLO and not the CC (assuming the tissue is projected onto the detector) since the breast is often better compressed on the CC projection. (Observation courtesy of Barbara Monsees, MD.)

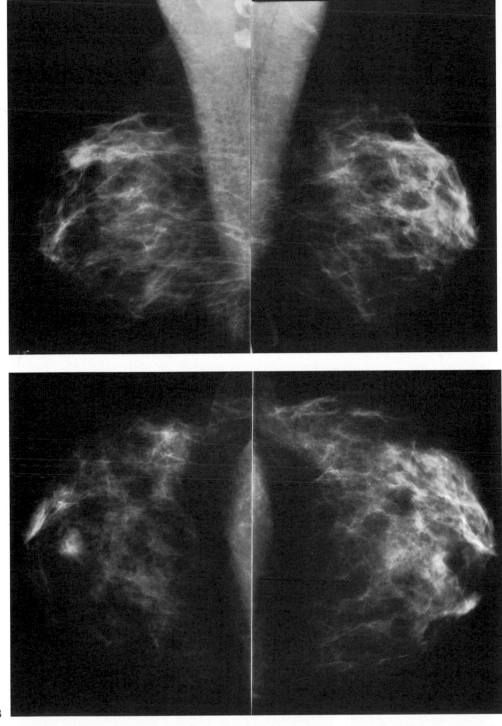

A

B

SC-3. A focal asymmetric density is evident in the anterior, superior, 12 o'clock region of the left breast on this screening study *(A)*. Additional imaging is indicated (BIRADS 0). Magnification views did not add any information *(B)*. The ultrasound study revealed a solid mass that proved to be a fibroadenoma on core needle biopsy. This was concordant with the imaging and no further evaluation was undertaken.

Teaching Point: The screening study is frequently insufficient to arrive at a final assessment without additional evaluation.

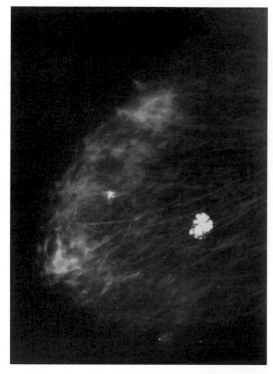

A

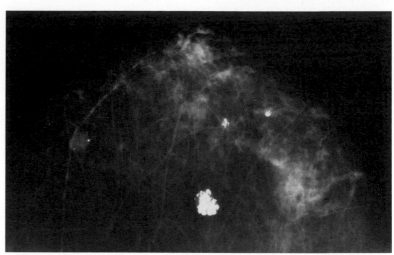

B

SC-4. Benign finding. This 69-year-old woman had a frozen left shoulder. On the MLO *(A)* and CC *(B)* projections there are large "popcorn"-like calcifications indicating benign, involuting fibroadenomas (BIRADS 2).

Teaching Point: If the finding is benign on the screening study, then no further evaluation is needed.

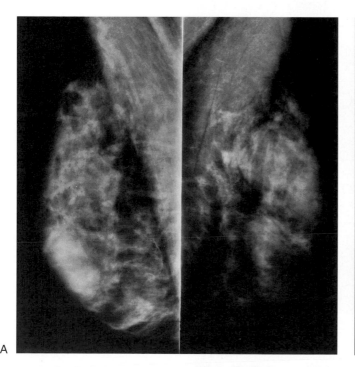

A

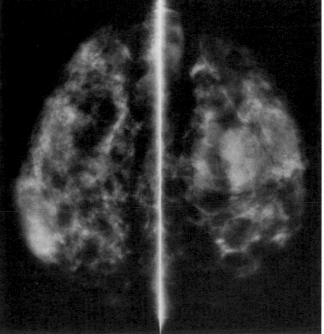

B

SC-5. Multiple rounded densities on screening mammograms. The rounded masses in the inferior, subareolar region on the left, and in the upper center of the right breast, as seen on the MLO *(A)* and CC *(B)* projections, proved to be cysts at ultrasound. Some would pass this on the screening study as multiple rounded densities that are likely benign (BIRADS 2). Others would place the patient into a follow-up category (BIRADS 3), while others would seek immediate additional evaluation (BIRADS 0).

Teaching Point: There is no uniform agreement as to how to manage every situation.

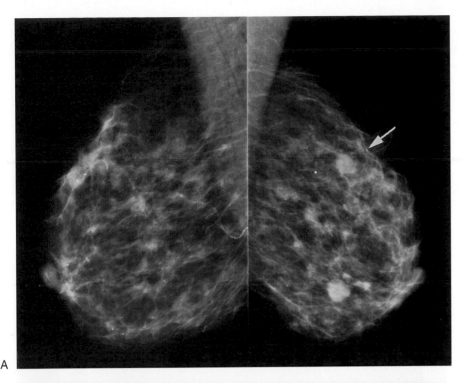

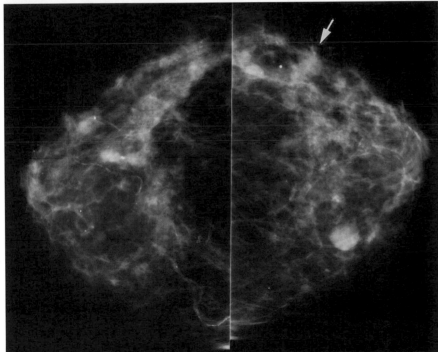

SC-6. Invasive cancer among multiple findings. The mass in the upper outer right breast *(arrows)* on the MLO *(A)* and CC *(B)* projections proved to be cancer, while all of the other rounded densities proved to be cysts.

Teaching Point: The "rule of multiplicity" (three or more of the same finding suggest benign processes) does not obviate the need to carefully evaluate the characteristics of each mass or set of calcifications when multiples are present. Cancer can exist alongside benign changes.

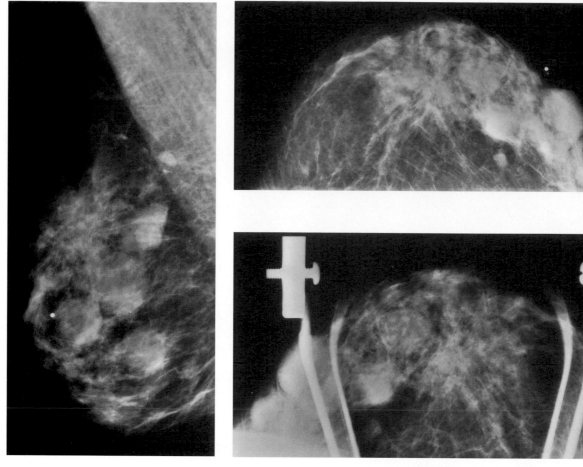

SC-7. Invasive breast cancer among cysts. The mammogram was obtained in the MLO *(A)* and CC *(B)* projections for the palpable cyst in the lateral left breast (marked with a *"BB"*). The spiculated architectural distortion in the anterior 12 o'clock left breast proved to be an occult invasive ductal carcinoma. Even on the spot compression view in the CC projection *(C)*, the lesion is fairly subtle.

Teaching Point: Avoid the "instant happiness" syndrome. Even though multiple rounded densities are almost always benign, the observer needs to search for lesions "in between."

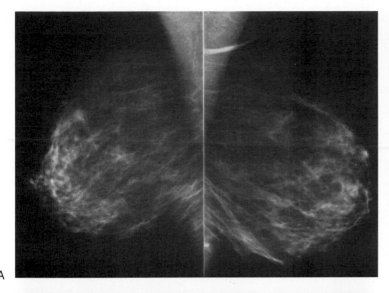

A

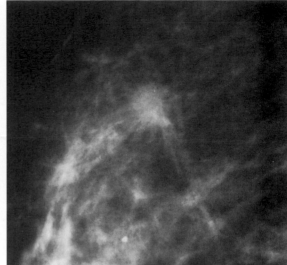

C

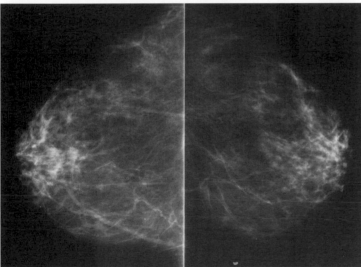

B

SC-8. Don't forget to look for **focal asymmetric density.** There is a focal asymmetric density that projects over the anterior, upper left breast on the MLO *(A)* that is much less apparent on the CC *(B)*. Closer inspection *(C)* reveals an irregular, spiculated mass (BI-RADS 5) that proved to be an invasive ductal carcinoma.

Teaching Points: 1. The benefit from screening comes with finding very small, early stage cancers. 2. It is not always necessary to recall a patient for additional evaluation to make a confident assessment as long as the lesion is confidently seen on the two projections.

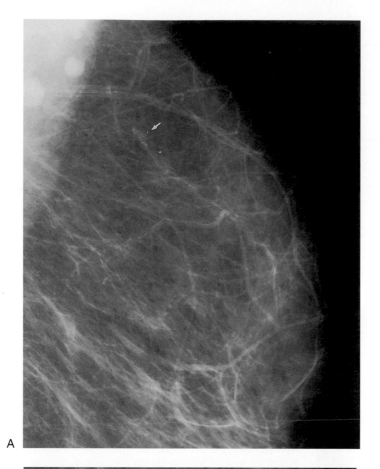

A

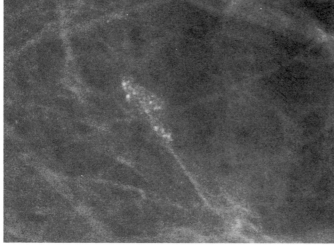

B

SC-9. Calcifications of ductal carcinoma *in situ* (DCIS). Calcifications such as these seen on the MLO *(A)* and enlarged MLO *(B)* should raise a high index of suspicion (BIRADS 4). These proved to be due to ductal carcinoma *in situ.* Calcifications are the earliest indication of breast cancer.

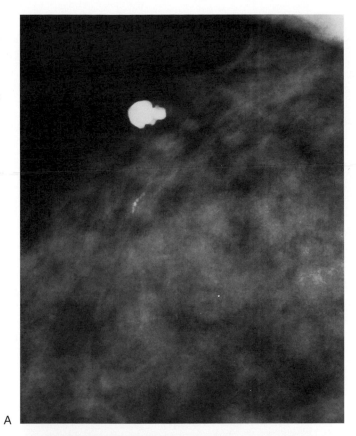

A

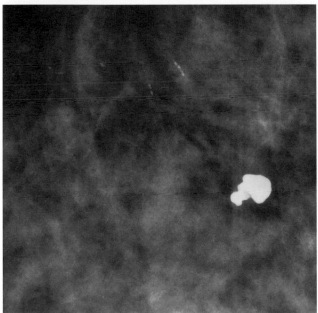

B

SC-10. Calcifications in intraductal carcinoma with invasion. These calcifications, in linear distributions, seen on the enlarged MLO *(A)* and CC *(B)* on the screening study proved to be in high-grade DCIS that was associated with a mammographically occult, poorly differentiated invasive breast cancer.

Teaching Points: 1. Calcifications, associated with breast cancer, do not always indicate an early-stage lesion. 2. Calcifications are important, but don't forget to look carefully for masses and areas of architectural distortion since invasive cancers are much more likely to reach a level of lethality earlier than *in situ* cancer.

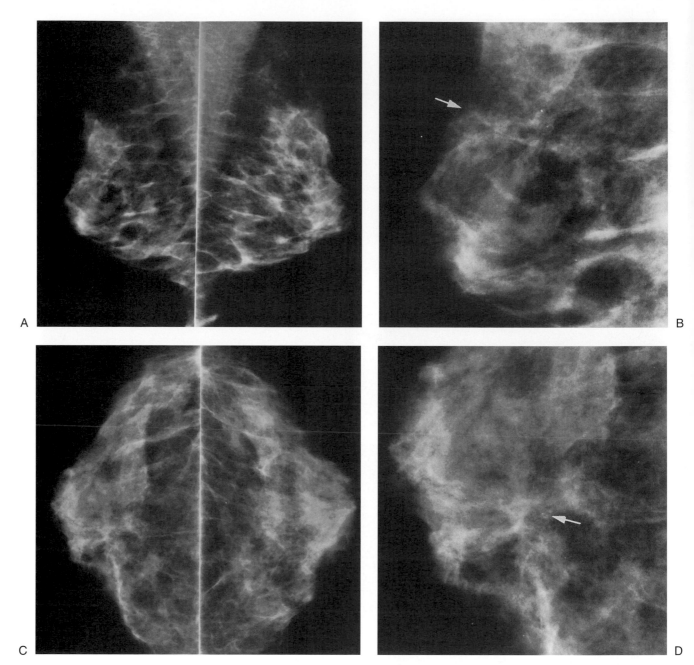

SC-11. Don't forget architectural distortion. Subtle areas of architectural distortion can be overlooked. This invasive cancer was extremely subtle on the MLO *(A)* and enlarged MLO *(B)*. It was a little more prominent on the CC *(C)* and enlarged CC *(D)* projections.

Teaching Point: Cancer can manifest itself as calcifications, a focal asymmetric density, a true mass, or as architectural distortion.

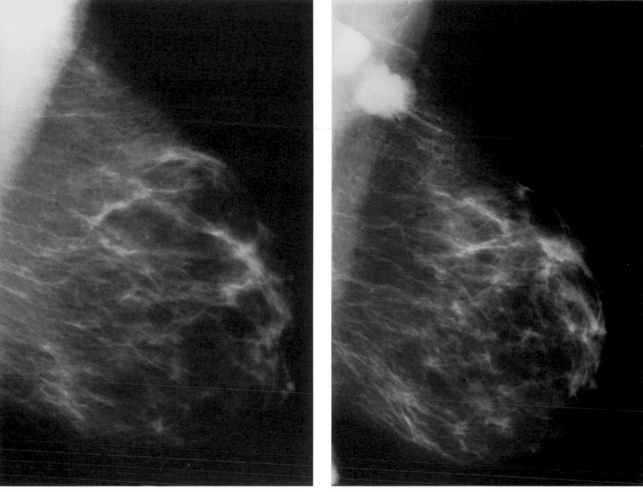

A   B

SC-12. The time between screens is not trivial. This woman was 49 years old when she had this mammogram *(A)*. She did not return for another 2 years and 3 months, by which time her invasive breast cancer had grown to 2.5 cm and she had metastatic disease to her axillary lymph nodes *(B)*.

Teaching Point: It is not merely being screened that is important. Too long a time between screens can mean that a cancer grows too large to be cured.

Section II:
Calcifications on Mammograms

If evaluated in detail, virtually every breast will contain one or more calcifications. The vast majority of calcifications are due to benign processes. The assessment of calcium deposits is assisted by using magnification mammography. When further evaluation is indicated, based on the screening study, we obtain magnification images of the calcifications to improve our ability to determine their number, extent, and morphology. We routinely obtain a horizontal beam, magnification lateral projection as one of the views along with a magnification CC (craniocaudal), since these permit high spatial resolution for morphologic assessment, and the horizontal beam image will provide information as to whether or not we are dealing with benign "milk of calcium" (see below).

Some have argued that there has been too much emphasis on calcifications, because, when associated with malignancy, they almost always indicate intraductal cancer that may not be a threat for many years. However, one researcher has found that, if left alone, even the calcifications associated with low-grade ductal carcinoma *in situ* (DCIS) may become advanced invasive cancers 10 to 20 years later (personal communication). This has been confirmed by David Page in a follow-up of women with low-grade DCIS whose diagnosis was initially missed (so that they were incompletely treated). Not only did 9 out of 28 women (32%) develop recurrences (7 were invasive), but 5 women (18%) eventually died from their breast cancers. In order to try to save lives from cancers that threaten the individual in the near term, screening must detect the small invasive cancers (masses and architectural distortion) that may become lethal (successfully metastatic) over the short term, but finding DCIS will likely reduce the risk of mortality in the long term.

There has been a recent effort to differentiate the forms of DCIS that appear to have different natural histories, and they are thus classified as well differentiated, moderately well differentiated, or poorly differentiated. In an effort to elevate the role of mammography, many have suggested that histology can be deduced from mammographic findings. We have not been able to show that different forms of DCIS can be predicted from their mammographic appearance. Although, in general, trying to guess histology from a mammogram is merely speculation, there are, however, some types of calcifications that are fairly predictive on a mammogram and can be described with certainty. [See *Breast Imaging, Second Edition,* pp.315–338.]

PROCESS-SPECIFIC CALCIFICATIONS AND TYPICALLY BENIGN CALCIFICATIONS

Skin Calcifications

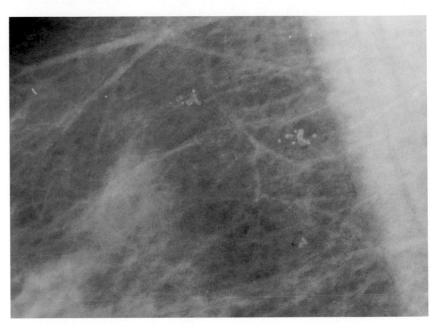

C-1. Skin calcifications. These deposits have the characteristic lucent centers with geographic shapes. No further evaluation is needed. [See *Breast Imaging, Second Edition,* pp. 319–321.]

Vascular Calcifications

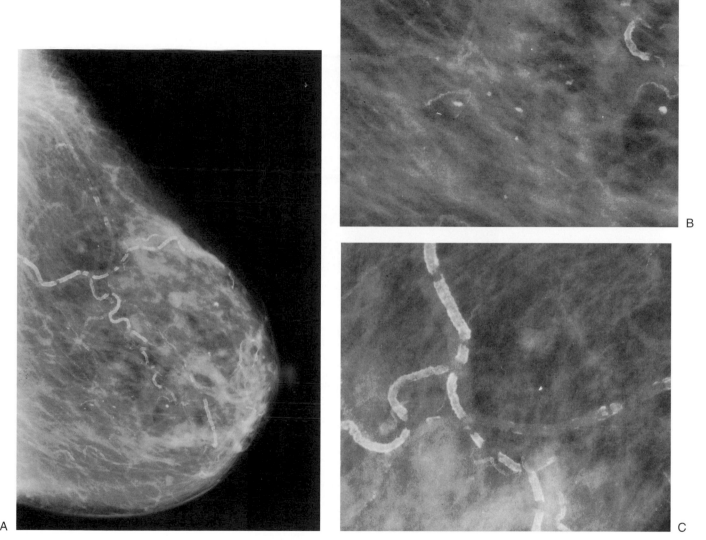

A

B

C

C-2. Vascular calcifications. The parallel, curvilinear calcifications are typical vascular calcifications *(A)*. Both large and small vessel calcifications are seen on this photographic enlargement *(B)*. Cancer calcifications do not form parallel deposits. As with most arterial deposits, these are calcifications in the intima of the arterial wall seen in this enlargement in a second patient *(C)*. [See *Breast Imaging, Second Edition,* pp. 317–319, 324.]

Teaching Point: Parallel calcifications conforming to the walls of a tubular structure are never due to cancer, but are vascular.

Large Coarse "Popcorn"-Shaped Calcifications

[See *Breast Imaging, Second Edition*, p. 325]

There is no absolute definition of what constitutes a coarse calcification. They are generally larger than 1 mm and frequently several millimeters to a centimeter or more in diameter. Coarse calcifications are almost always indicative of a benign process, but if finer, irregular, clustered calcifications are associated with some larger forms, the smaller calcifications should lead to earlier biopsy.

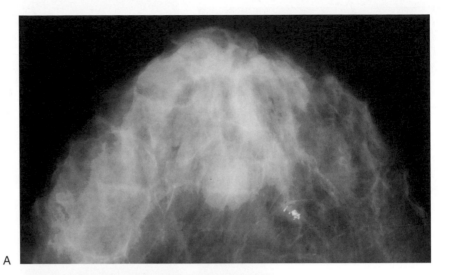

A

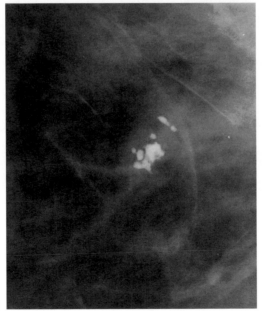

B

C-3. Involuting fibroadenoma. *(A)* These coarse calcifications, seen close up *(B)*, appear to be in the center of a vague mass. Their size and central location in the mass ensure the diagnosis of a benign, involuting fibroadenoma.

Teaching Point: Large calcifications in the center of a mass virtually always indicate an involuting fibroadenoma.

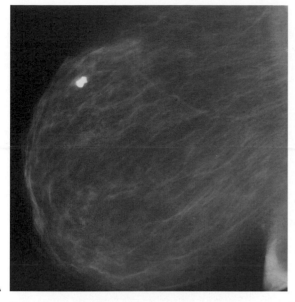
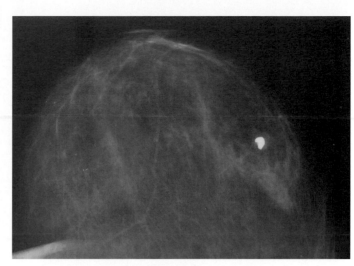

A   B

C-4. Involuted fibroadenoma. The large, coarse calcification in the upper *(A)* outer *(B)* left breast is consistent with an involuted fibroadenoma.

Teaching Point: Large, irregularly shaped calcifications are almost always involuted fibroadenomas.

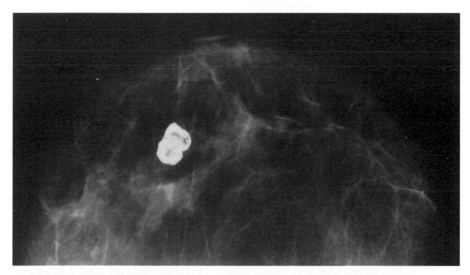

C-5. Involuted fibroadenoma. This large "popcorn"-shaped calcification was hard on clinical breast examination, but a biopsy is not required. This is the typical appearance of an involuted fibroadenoma.

Teaching Point: Large "popcorn"-shaped calcifications are always benign.

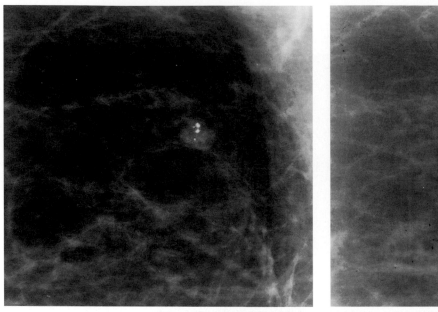
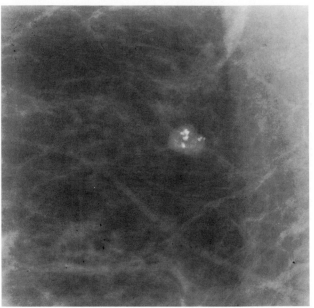

A   B

C-6. Progressive involution of a fibroadenoma. There are coarse calcifications in the lobulated mass deep in the left breast *(A)*. A year later *(B)*, the calcifications in this fibroadenoma have increased in number and are larger. No further investigation is needed.

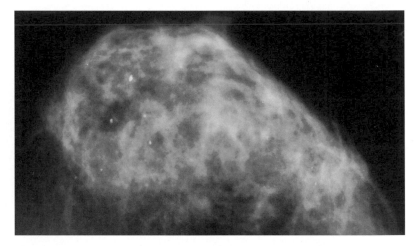

C-7. Nonspecific coarse calcifications are benign. The coarse calcifications seen on this craniocaudal projection are sufficiently large that no further investigation is required. They likely represent irregularly calcified debris in ectatic ducts.

Rod-Shaped "Secretory" Calcifications and Linear Calcifications

[See *Breast Imaging, Second Edition,* p. 325]

Large, rod-shaped calcifications conforming to the lumen of a duct are benign if they are solid and continuous without branching forms and are more than 0.5 mm in diameter. They are the result of calcification of debris that has collected in the duct. The process has been termed "secretory disease." Benign, rod-shaped calcifications may also have lucent centers.

Linear calcifications, in general, form in the lumen of the duct, which molds them to their shape. Other linear calcifications appear in parallel and are vascular in location.

Linear calcifications, however, that are composed of very small particles and form in an interrupted pattern that is linear in distribution, especially with branching forms, should be considered suspicious.

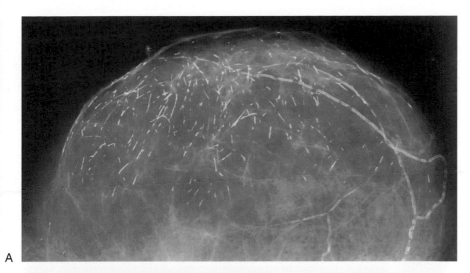

A

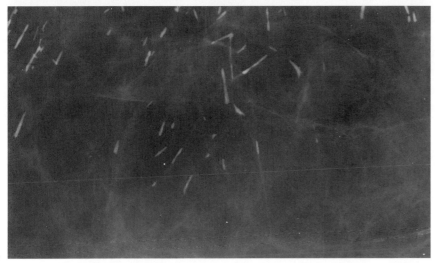

B

C-8. Rod-shaped calcifications. These thick (greater than 0.5 mm in diameter), rod-shaped calcifications *(A)*, oriented along duct lines that are shown enlarged *(B)*, are typical of benign "secretory" deposits and should not elicit any concern.

Teaching Point: If the rods are solid, then they represent benign secretory disease and no further investigation is needed. If they are made up of smaller particles, then the possibility of ductal carcinoma *in situ* should be considered.

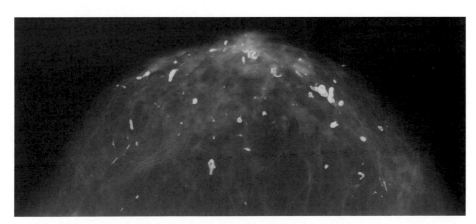

C-9. Lucent-centered rods are also benign deposits. These large, dense, lucent-centered, rod-shaped calcifications are believed to represent another form of benign secretory disease.

Round, Smooth Calcifications

[See *Breast Imaging, Second Edition,* pp. 325–326.]

Solid round, smooth calcifications are fairly common and likely represent areas of fat necrosis or debris in ducts. When individual, or in groups of two to four, they are of no concern. Clustered (five or more in 1 cm³ of tissue), solid, round, smooth calcifications that are 1 mm or smaller (microcalcifications) are fairly uncommon. If they form a cluster, but are round and regular on magnification imaging, Sickles' data suggest that they can be safely followed.

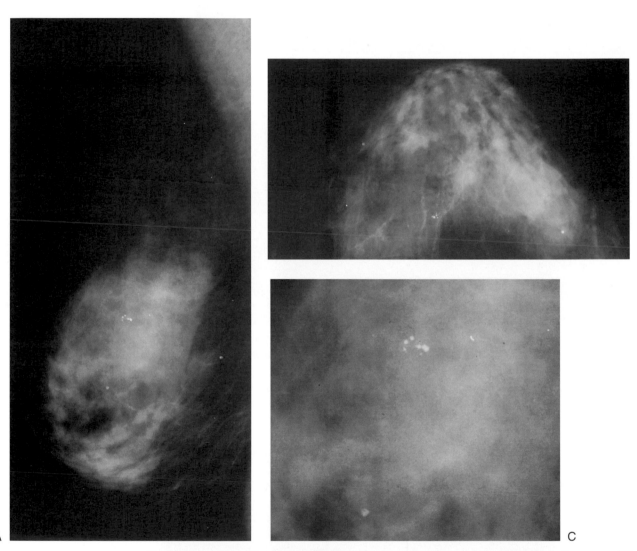

C-10. Round calcifications in fibrous stroma. *(A)* Clustered calcifications in the upper *(B)* central portion of the breast, photographically enlarged *(C)*, are round and regular, with the exception of a few pleomorphic forms. As a consequence of the latter, a biopsy was performed and the calcifications proved to be in an area of benign fibrosis.

Teaching Point: Round, smooth calcifications are almost always due to benign processes and are, in our experience, generally in the breast stroma.

C-11. Benign round and regular calcifications. These calcifications, seen on magnification mammography, are round and regular. They have been stable for over 5 years and are due to a benign process.

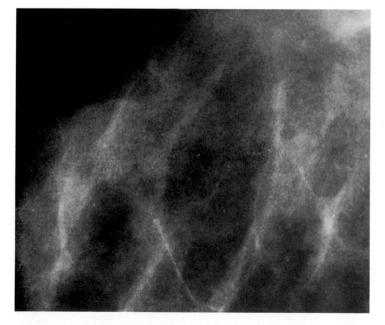

C-12. These round, regular **punctate calcifications** on magnification mammography were sampled because of their segmental distribution and were found to be in the fibrous stroma of the breast. It is unclear how or why they form. Perhaps they develop in "burned out" lobules.

Teaching Point: Sickles' data suggest that if calcifications are smooth, round, and regular, then short-interval follow-up is reasonable since the likelihood of cancer is less than 2%.

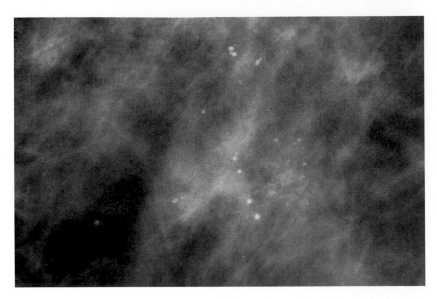

C-13. Benign round and regular calcifications. These calcifications are each very round and smooth. They have remained unchanged for over 5 years.

Lucent-Centered Calcifications

[See *Breast Imaging, Second Edition,* p. 326]

Lucent-centered calcifications are always benign and should not cause concern. They may represent secretory deposits, areas of fat necrosis, or may be in the skin and not in the breast itself.

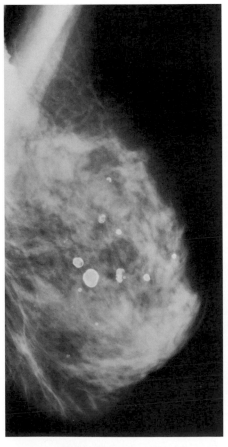

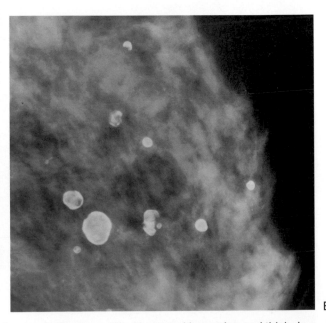

C-14. Fat necrosis. Numerous large calcifications *(A)* with central lucencies and thick rims in the right breast are most likely related to areas of fat necrosis and are benign. They are shown enlarged *(B).*

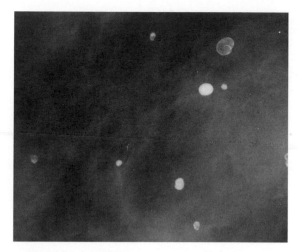

C-15. Benign calcifications. These lucent-centered deposits are due to benign processes. They are likely found in debris in ducts.

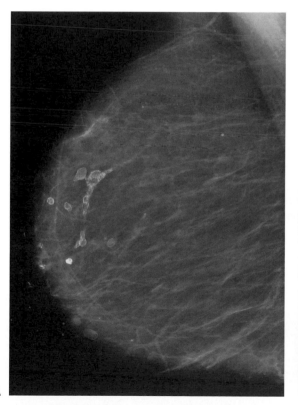

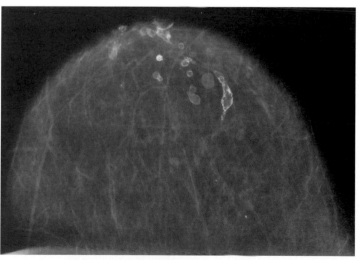

A   B

C-16. Fat necrosis from a seatbelt injury. These large, lucent-centered calcifications on the MLO *(A)* and CC *(B)* projections were due to fat necrosis from wearing a seatbelt that compressed the breast during an automobile collision.

Teaching Point: One response to fat necrosis is the "walling off" of the dead fat cells by the tissue response and calcification of the walled off, gelatinized fat.

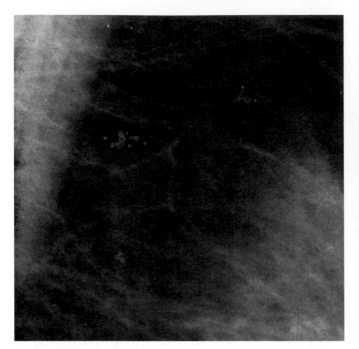

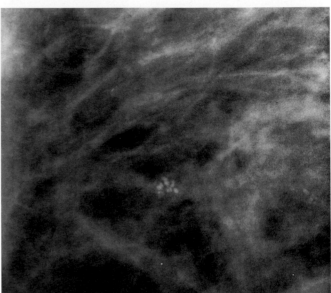

C-17. Skin calcifications. Skin calcifications are almost always lucent centered, as are these benign dermal deposits.

Teaching Point: Lucent-centered calcifications that have geometric shapes are almost always benign deposits in the skin.

C-18. Skin calcifications. These calcifications were initially thought to be pleomorphic and suspicious. Closer inspection reveals that many have lucent centers, and they were shown to be in the skin.

Teaching Point: Lucent-centered calcifications are almost invariably due to benign processes and are only coincidentally found in association with breast cancer.

Rim or Eggshell Calcifications

[See *Breast Imaging, Second Edition,* pp. 326–328.]

Calcifications conforming to the walls of a sphere are virtually always due to benign processes. When these are extremely thin they are termed "eggshell." Eggshell calcifications almost invariably represent calcification in the wall of a cyst. On occasion, involuting fibroadenomas can also give rise to thin, rimlike deposits. Fat necrosis, too, may result in these deposits, although generally it causes the thick, spherical calcifications described in the preceding section.

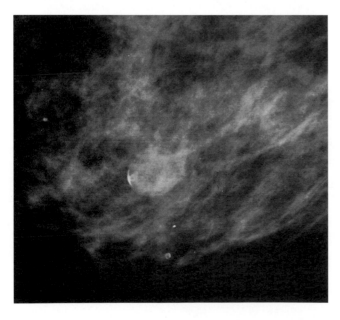

C-19. Cyst wall, "eggshell" calcifications. These rim-like deposits at the anterior periphery of a mass are typical of calcification in the wall of a cyst, and no further evaluation is necessary.

Teaching Point: Cyst-wall calcifications tend to be very fine and curvilinear.

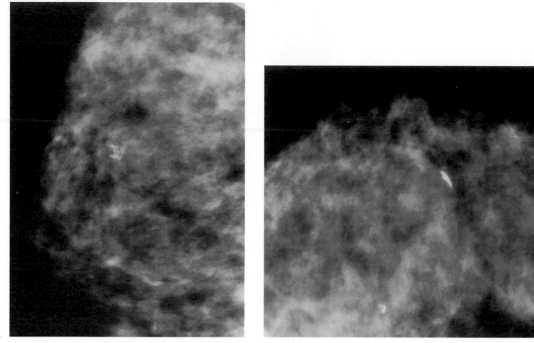

A   B

C-20. Calcifications in a cyst wall. These calcifications are forming a curvilinear plaque conforming to the rim of a spherical structure on the magnification lateral *(A)* and CC *(B)* projections. They are likely fixed deposits in, or adherent to, the wall of a cyst.

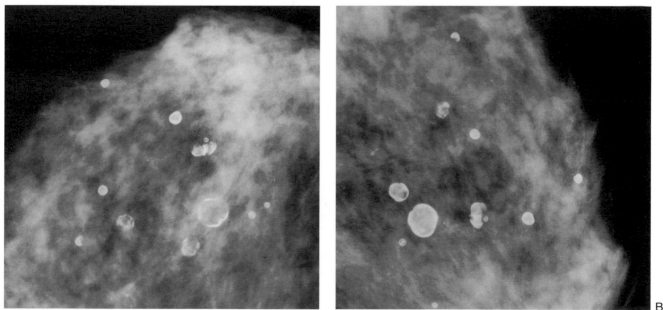

A   B

C-21. Progressive rim calcifications probably due to fat necrosis. There are round densities with thick calcifications that have formed, presumably in the walls *(A)*, but there are several spheres that have finer deposits. The latter become progressively thicker *(B)*. These are probably all areas of fat necrosis.

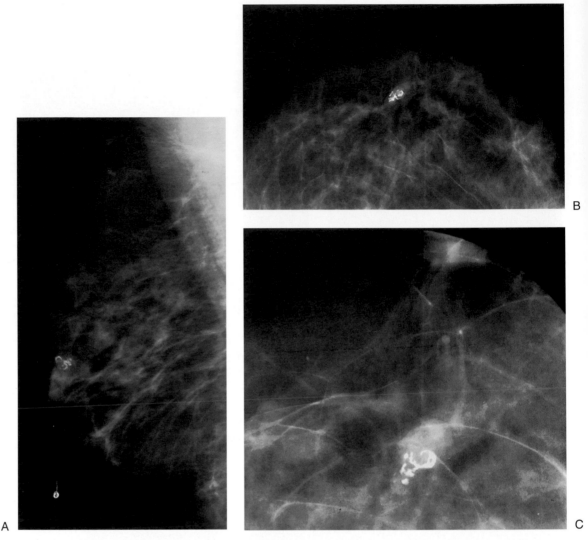

C-22. Atypical rim calcifications associated with a probable intraductal papilloma. Most rim calcifications form in or on the wall of a spherical lesion. These calcifications in the subareolar region on the MLO *(A)* and CC *(B)* projections can be seen on magnification *(C)* to be somewhat irregular "rim-like" deposits associated with a lobulated mass whose axis is directed toward the nipple. These have remained unchanged over more than 5 years and are consistent with calcifications of an intraductal papilloma.

Teaching Point: Rim calcifications associated with a probable intraductal mass close to the nipple are likely delineating a benign, intraductal papilloma.

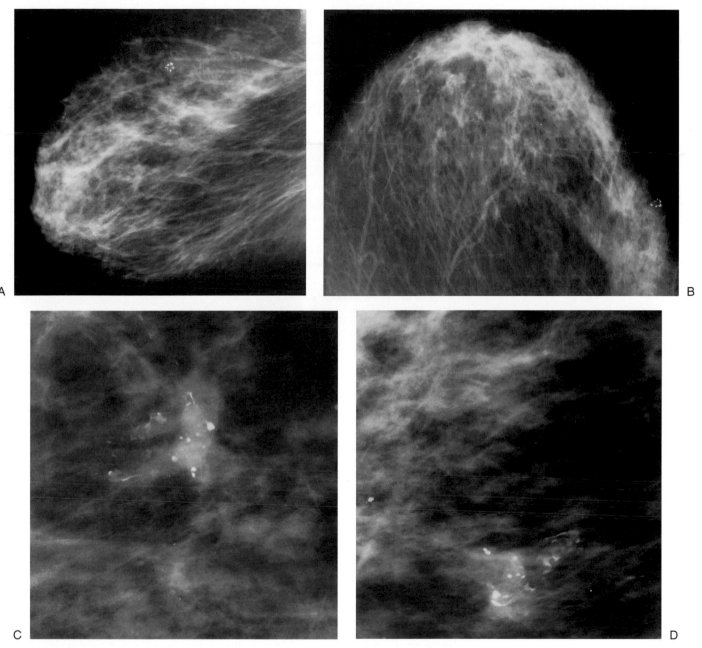

C-23. Rim calcifications formed along this lobulated, elongated density seen on the MLO *(A)*, CC *(B)*, straight lateral magnification *(C)*, and CC magnification views *(D)*. The patient insisted on a biopsy, which revealed a **papilloma**. The other group of calcifications in the upper outer portion of the left breast is likely an involuting fibroadenoma.

Teaching Point: Rim calcifications virtually always suggest a benign tumor. Cancer necroses internally. Papillomas rarely calcify. When they do, it is likely due to ischemia to the distal tissues nourished by the fibrovascular stalk. This probably explains why the calcifications appear at the ends of the fronds as reflected in the mammographic appearance.

Milk of Calcium

[See *Breast Imaging, Second Edition,* p. 328]

Calcium that precipitates in cysts can form a thin deposit of powder that layers in the dependent portion of the cyst. This has the typical crescent shape in the horizontal beam lateral projection and an amorphous appearance in the craniocaudal projection. Calcium can also form into round ball-shaped particles or it can become concretions in the cyst.

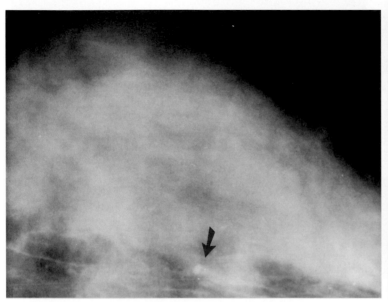
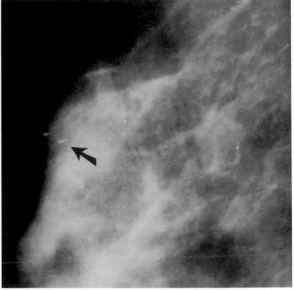

A   B

C-24. Milk of calcium. These calcifications appear to be curvilinear, concave up on the straight lateral projection *(A)* and amorphous on the CC projection *(B)*. These can only represent precipitated calcium in small cysts.

Teaching Point: Milk-of-calcium calcifications are viewed by most as evidence of benign cystic changes.

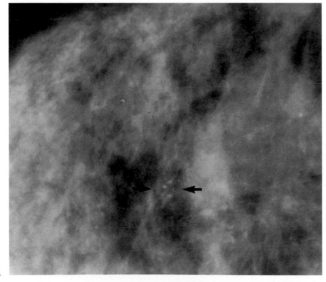
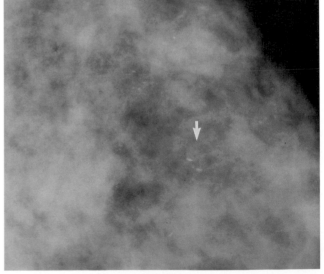

A   B

C-25. Milk of calcium. These calcifications are also precipitated calcifications, seen as amorphous calcifications on the CC *(A)* projection and curvilinear, concave up on the horizontal beam lateral projection *(B)*. No further evaluation is needed.

Suture Calcifications

[See *Breast Imaging, Second Edition*, p. 329]

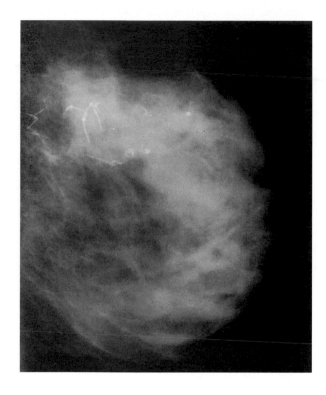

C-26. Suture calcifications. Calcifications that are in an area of previous surgery, as here, and are shaped like knots or sutures, are almost certainly due to calcified suture material. This is most common if the patient has been irradiated, or a reduction mammoplasty has been performed.

Dystrophic Calcifications

[See *Breast Imaging, Second Edition*, p. 329]

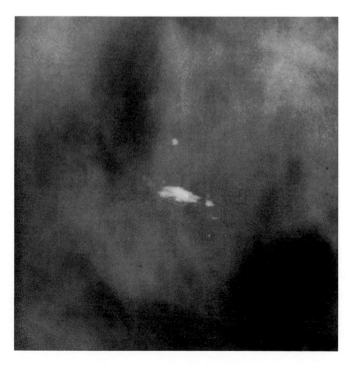

C-27. Dystrophic calcifications. These large, irregularly shaped calcifications are nonspecific. They have not changed in over 5 years, and likely represent "dystrophic deposits."

Teaching Point: Dystrophic calcifications usually are seen following surgery and irradiation. Sometimes they occur in otherwise healthy breast tissue.

Punctate Calcifications

[See *Breast Imaging, Second Edition,* p. 332.]

Punctate calcifications are very small, "pinpoint" (under 0.5 mm) calcifications that are, despite their small size, very sharply defined. In our experience they are often due to a benign process, but not infrequently they form in association with cancer.

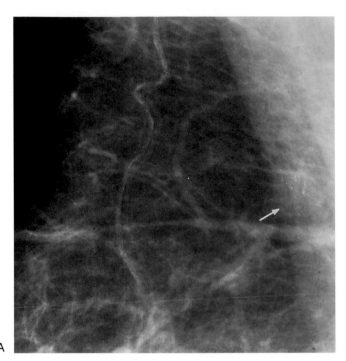
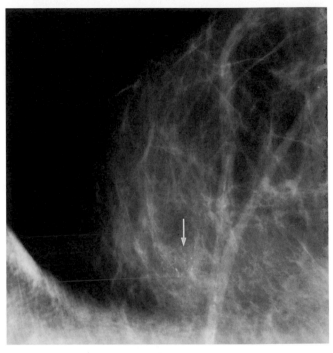

A   B

C-28. Punctate pseudocalcifications in a skin lesion. The tiny (0.2–0.3 mm) particles *(arrows)* seen on the lateral *(A)* and CC *(B)* projections are typical in appearance for "punctate" calcifications. They turned out, however, to be powder particles trapped in the irregular surface of a skin lesion.

Teaching Point: Skin calcifications and contaminants may appear as punctate deposits.

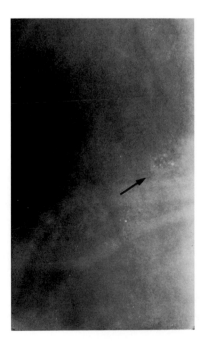

C-29. Sclerosing adenosis. Since sclerosing adenosis causes elongation and thinning of the lobular acini, it is not surprising that calcifications that form in those acini are very small. However, since the diagnosis could not be definitively made from the mammogram, a biopsy confirmed the diagnosis.

Teaching Point: Although the diagnosis of sclerosing adenosis can be suggested, it is safer to biopsy a cluster like this.

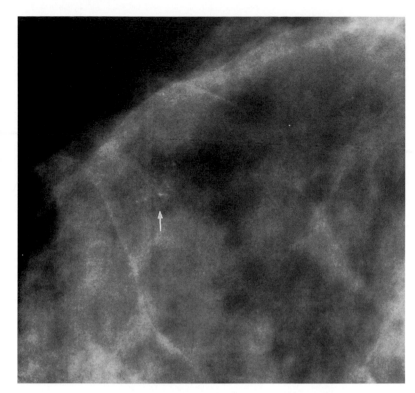

C-30. Sclerosing adenosis. These punctate calcifications were localized and biopsied and found to be in sclerosing adenosis.

Teaching Point: Sometimes you just can't tell (see C-31).

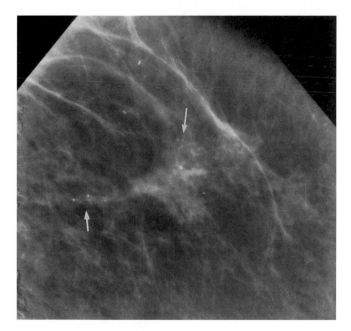

C-31. Punctate calcifications forming in DCIS. These punctate calcifications are very similar to those in C-30, but they were formed in DCIS.

Teaching Point: Sometimes you just can't tell benign calcifications from those caused by a malignancy.

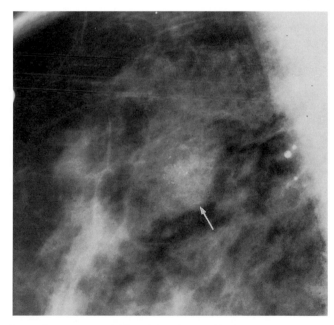

C-32. Punctate calcifications formed in intraductal carcinoma. This is a magnification view. The particles are each 0.2 to 0.3 mm in diameter.

Teaching Point: Cancer can produce very small but relatively dense calcifications.

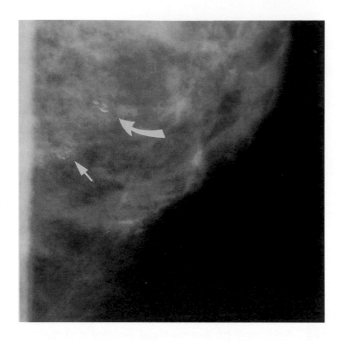

C-33. Punctate calcifications in DCIS beside benign milk of calcium. The curvilinear calcifications are due to benign milk of calcium *(curved arrow)*. The punctate calcifications were in DCIS.

Teaching Point: Avoid the "instant happiness" syndrome. Keep looking.

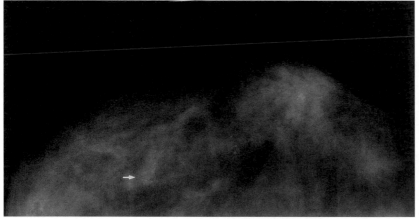

A

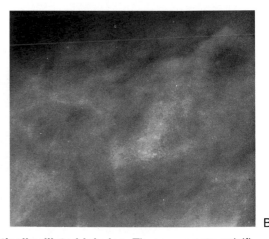

B

C-34. Benign calcifications in microcystically dilated lobules. These punctate calcifications on the CC projection *(A)* and enlarged *(B)* were in benign lobular acini.

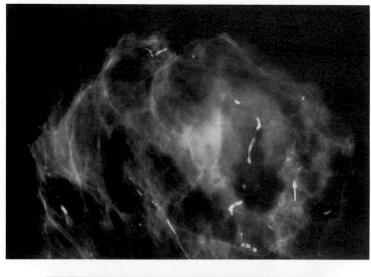

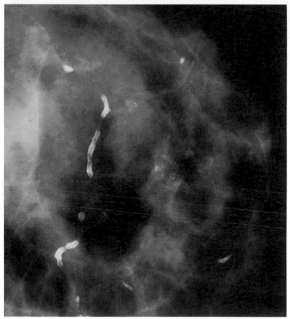

C-35. Punctate calcifications in DCIS. The innumerable punctate deposits seen on the CC projection *(A)* and enlarged *(B)* proved to be in DCIS.

Teaching Point: You often can't differentiate calcifications that are due to a benign process from those due to a malignant process.

INDETERMINATE AND NONSPECIFIC CALCIFICATIONS

[See *Breast Imaging, Second Edition,* p. 332.]

Amorphous Calcifications

Amorphous calcifications have basically round shapes, but their edges are fuzzy.

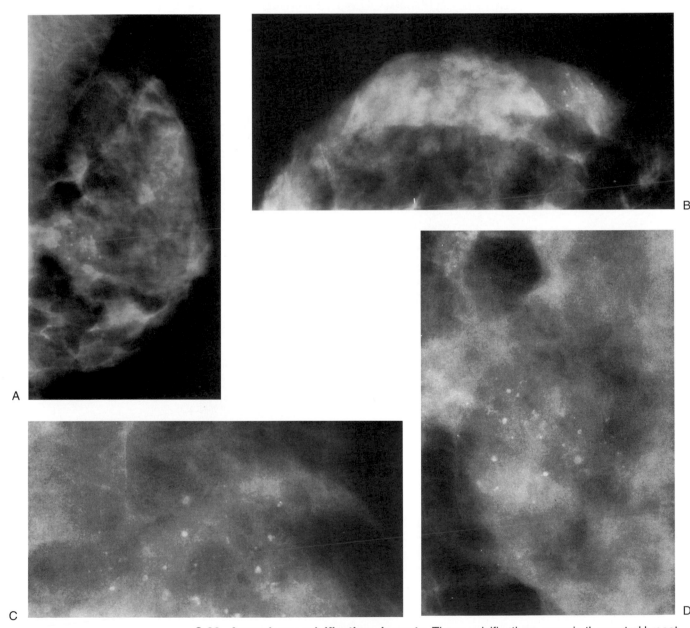

C-36. Amorphous calcifications in cysts. These calcifications, seen in the central breast on the MLO *(A)*, and medially on the CC *(B)*, are amorphous on the magnification view *(C)*. They did not layer dependently on the lateral *(D)*. They were biopsied because the patient wished certainty, and they proved to be calcium deposits in small cysts.

Teaching Point: Amorphous calcifications are likely a form of precipitated calcium that is not mobile like milk of calcium, but forms agglomerations in small cysts.

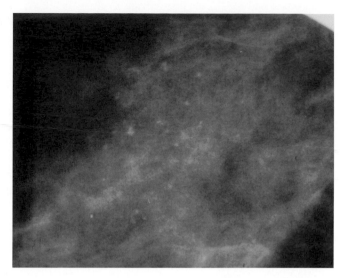

C-37. Calcium in microcysts. These vague, amorphous calcifications on magnification mammography proved to be in small cysts and the fibrous stroma (presumably "burned-out" lobules). Their small size and heterogeneous forms caused suspicion and a biopsy.

Teaching Point: Amorphous calcifications are almost always associated with microcysts. The mixture of cyst fluid and calcium particles likely accounts for their fuzzy appearance.

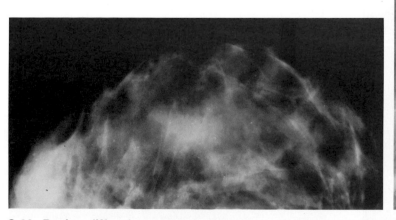

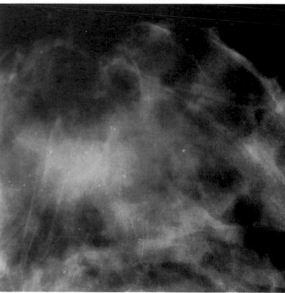

A

B

C-38. Benign diffusely scattered, amorphous calcifications. This 47-year-old woman has calcifications that are diffusely scattered in her right breast on this CC projection *(A)*. Close inspection *(B)* reveals the amorphous morphology of the individual particles. They have been stable for 7 years.

Teaching Point: Diffusely scattered calcifications (see below) are usually amorphous and virtually always benign.

INCREASED PROBABILITY OF MALIGNANCY

[See *Breast Imaging, Second Edition,* pp. 333–334.]

Pleomorphic Calcifications

Calcifications associated with cancer are virtually always pleomorphic. The greater the heterogeneity of the shapes of the individual deposits, the greater the likelihood of cancer. Benign lesions can also produce heterogeneous deposits, but they tend to form more regular shapes. Magnification mammography will frequently give a better appreciation of the number, morphology, and distribution of the particles. Nevertheless, it is often impossible to differentiate benign from malignant calcifications by mammography, and a biopsy is frequently required to distinguish the two.

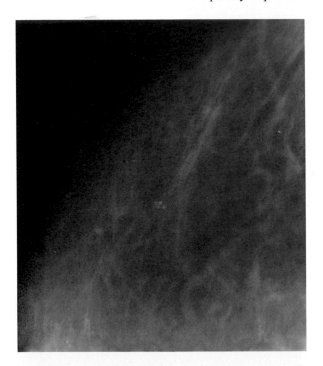

C-39. Skin calcifications. Occasionally skin calcifications are indistinguishable from intramammary deposits. These calcifications each measure 0.5 mm in diameter. Most skin calcifications have lucent centers, but on occasion they do not have this typical feature. A tangential projection proved that these were in the skin.

Teaching Point: Since most of the skin projects over the breast, skin calcifications are usually seen projecting over the breast. This diagnosis should be considered when the deposits are closely packed together and moderate in size (0.5–2.0 mm).

C-40. Pseudopleomorphic calcifications due to skin contamination. What appear to be pleomorphic and suspicious calcifications disappeared when the patient's skin was washed.

Teaching Point: Talc, zinc oxide, and antiperspirants on the skin can simulate clustered microcalcifications.

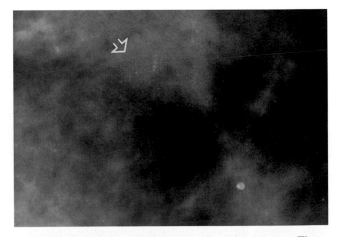

C-41. Pleomorphic calcifications in microcysts. These are indistinguishable from calcifications formed by DCIS. Biopsy proved that they were deposits in benign microcysts. The large spherical calcification is also benign.

Teaching Point: Clustered microcalcifications are frequently of uncertain etiology, and the diagnosis can only be made through a biopsy.

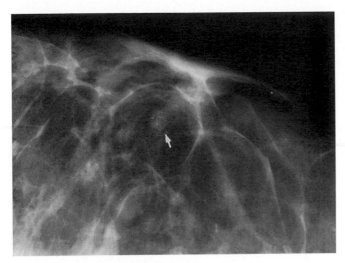

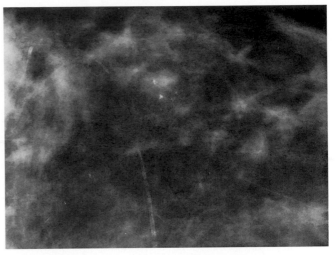

C-42. Calcifications in DCIS. This small mass with tiny calcifications could have been mistaken for a fibroadenoma, but it all proved to be DCIS.

Teaching Point: If the calcifications are small and pleomorphic, biopsy is warranted.

C-43. Sclerosing adenosis. These calcifications, seen on magnification mammography, were formed in benign sclerosing adenosis.

Teaching Point: Pleomorphism can occur with benign processes.

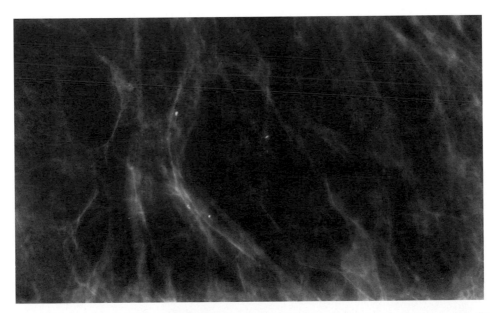

C-44. Poorly differentiated DCIS. Although some of the calcifications are somewhat dispersed over a 1- to 2-cm area, these calcifications met the criteria for a cluster of pleomorphic deposits and biopsy revealed DCIS.

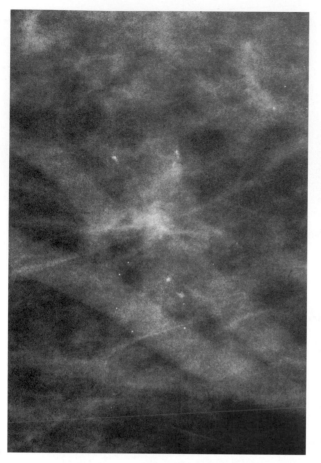

A

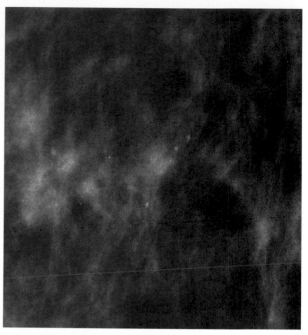

B

C-45. Poorly differentiated DCIS. This is another case of pleomorphic calcifications forming in DCIS seen on the magnification lateral *(A)* and CC *(B)*.

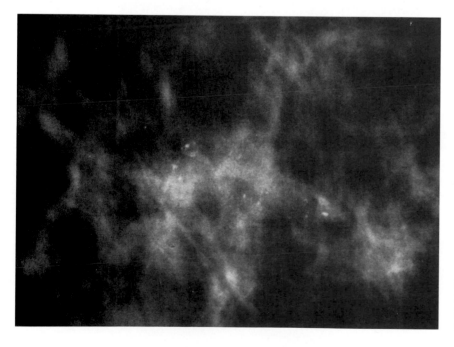

C-46. Poorly differentiated DCIS. Pleomorphic calcifications, as seen here on a magnification view, were due to poorly differentiated DCIS.

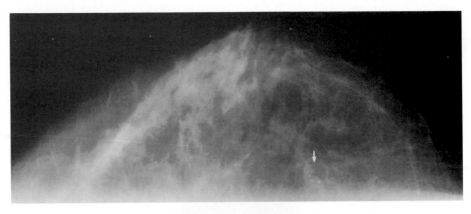

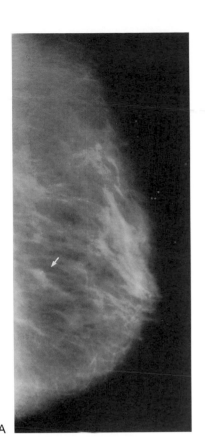

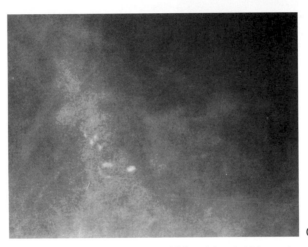

A

B

C

C-47. Peripheral duct papillomas. The calcifications seen in the middle of the right breast on the lateral mammogram *(A)* and the CC mammogram *(B)* and the photographically enlarged CC *(C)* are irregular in size and shape. Biopsy revealed a benign papilloma in a small duct.

Teaching Point: These calcifications are indistinguishable from those seen with some breast cancers. Some data suggest that peripheral duct papillomas represent a genetically "unstable epithelium" and an increased risk for cancer.

C-48. Poorly differentiated DCIS. These calcifications are at the edge of the parenchyma in a very dense breast of a 33-year-old woman with a nipple discharge. They proved to be in poorly differentiated DCIS.

C-49. Calcifications in DCIS. The pronounced variation in size and shape of the calcifications prompted a biopsy that revealed poorly differentiated DCIS.

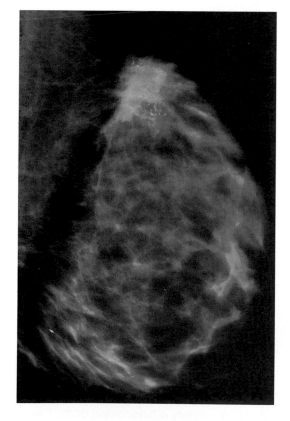

C-50. Pleomorphic calcifications associated with an invasive breast cancer. The visualization of this large, irregularly shaped, invasive breast cancer is not a triumph for mammography. However, it illustrates the association between invasive and intraductal carcinoma. The calcifications were due to high-grade DCIS. The invasive cancer was a high-grade invasive ductal carcinoma.

Teaching Points: 1. The calcifications associated with an invasive cancer are, almost always, in the intraductal portion of the tumor (they are rarely in just necrotic tissue in the center of a large cancer). This illustrates what is often the natural history of breast cancer. If DCIS is present for a long-enough period of time, an invasive clone may arise. Often the DCIS persists with the invasive cancer growing around it. At other times, the invasive cancer may obliterate the DCIS as it does the normal tissues. 2. The histologic grade of the invasive cancer is usually the same as the intraductal component.

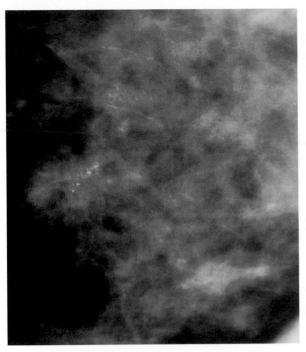 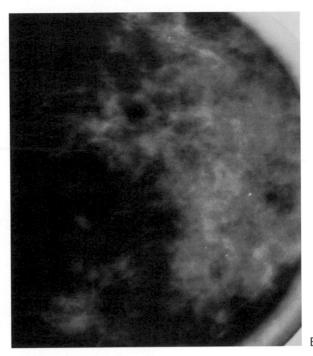

A   B

C-51. Calcifications due to DCIS associated with **invasive breast cancer.** These pleomorphic, clustered calcifications, seen on magnification straight lateral *(A)* and CC *(B)* views, were due to moderately differentiated DCIS. They were part of the intraductal component of what proved to be a 1.3-cm, moderately well differentiated, invasive breast cancer in a 53-year-old woman whose ten excised axillary lymph nodes were negative.

Teaching Points: 1. Calcifications associated with breast cancer are almost always in the intraductal component, but they do not always indicate only DCIS. 2. Generally, the differentiation of the DCIS is reflected in the grade of the invasive lesion, although some data suggest that, with time, poorly differentiated clones will eventually select themselves to dominate.

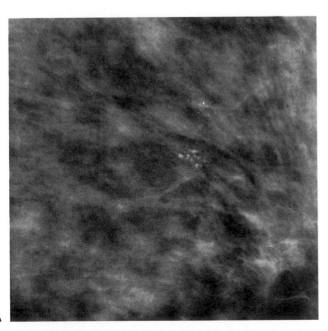 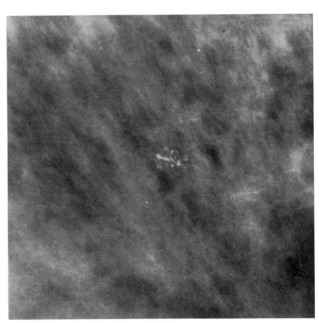

A   B

C-52. Mixed DCIS. This cluster of pleomorphic calcifications, as seen on the magnification straight lateral *(A)* and CC *(B)* views, proved to be a mixture of cribriform and micropapillary DCIS that also demonstrated comedonecrosis.

Teaching Point: Nature does not always cooperate. Different clones can form in the same lesion.

Fine, Linear Branching Calcifications

[See *Breast Imaging, Second Edition,* p. 334.]

Calcifications that appear to conform to a ductal distribution and are not the solid rods or lucent-centered calcifications of benign secretory deposits should be considered with a high degree of suspicion.

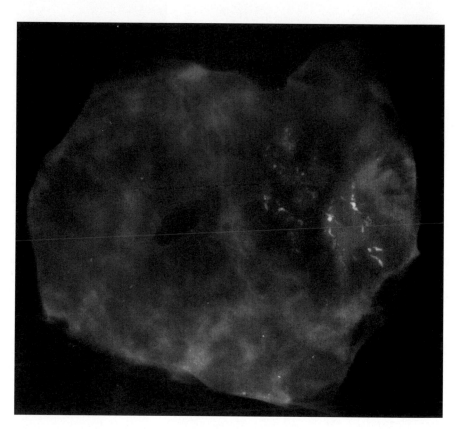

C-53. Specimen radiograph of DCIS calcifications. This specimen radiograph of poorly differentiated DCIS demonstrates the pleomorphic, fine, linear, branching pattern of calcifications that are quite characteristic of intraductal cancer.

Teaching Point: Unlike secretory calcifications that form continuous rod-shaped calcifications, the linear deposits in DCIS are, under close inspection, made up of numerous smaller particles.

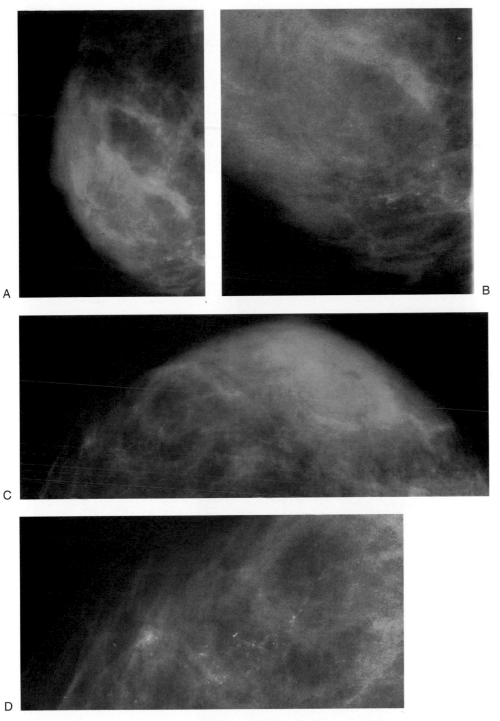

C-54. A linear, branching distribution of calcifications in DCIS. These calcifications seen in the lower left breast *(A)*, enlarged *(B)*, are fine, pleomorphic, and in a linear branching distribution as seen in the craniocaudal view *(C)* and enlarged *(D)* CC projection. The distribution is due to their formation in ducts that are filled with tumor cells, many of which are necrotic and calcified.

Teaching Point: Fine calcifications in a linear, branching pattern are almost always an indication of intraductal carcinoma.

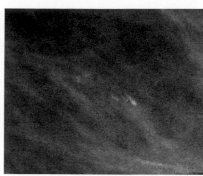

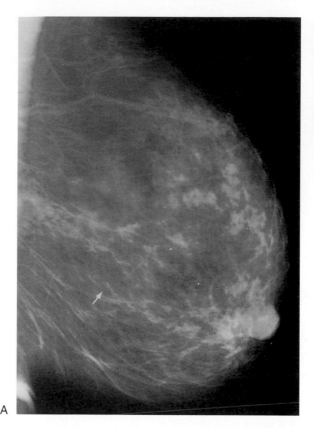

A

C-55. Intraductal carcinoma. These fine calcifications forming a linear pattern *(A)* are, on closer inspection, numerous tiny particles in a linear distribution *(B)*. These proved to be a small duct segment involved with DCIS.

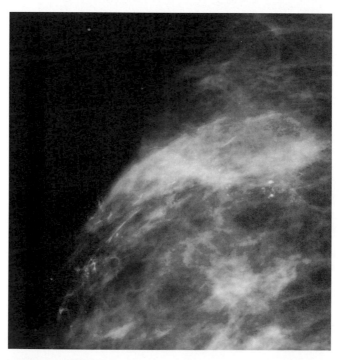

C-56. Fine, linear branching calcifications of DCIS. This pattern of fine calcifications is almost diagnostic of DCIS.

Teaching Point: Fine linear calcifications in an interrupted pattern are highly suspicious.

DISTRIBUTION PATTERNS OF CALCIFICATIONS

[See *Breast Imaging, Second Edition,* p. 334.]

Clustered Microcalcifications

BIRADS suggests that the term *clustered microcalcifications* should not, necessarily, connote a likely malignant process. This is a general category of very small deposits, many of which are due to benign processes. Although thresholds vary, most studies suggest that five or more small (under 0.5 mm) calcifications in 1 cm^3 of breast tissue constitute a "cluster" and warrant careful evaluation. Although cancer associated calcifications must start at some point, it is extremely rare for a malignancy to be detected because of fewer than five calcifications. Calcifications that are very fine (less than 0.5 mm in diameter), and aligned in a "dot-dash" or branching pattern, should be considered especially suspicious for intraductal malignancy even if there are fewer than five deposits.

The greater the number of small calcifications, and the greater the heterogeneity of their shapes and sizes, the more suspicious they become. Calcifications associated with malignancy are generally under 0.5 mm in diameter and almost always under 1 mm. Nevertheless, larger calcifications can be seen in association with smaller deposits, and a lesion should be judged by the smallest, not the largest, calcifications. Most clustered microcalcifications, however, are due to benign processes.

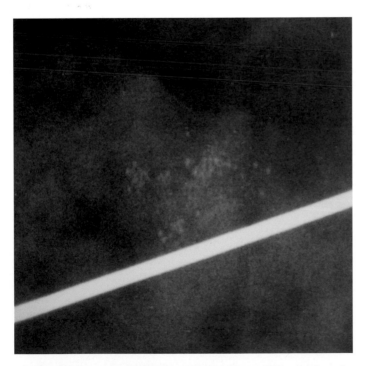

C-57. Benign pleomorphic calcifications. This cluster of calcifications, seen on this specimen radiograph, is pleomorphic, and the calcifications are innumerable, yet they were due to an atypical hyperplasia and were found in the acini of lobules.

Teaching Point: Not all pleomorphic, clustered calcifications are due to cancer. This is why biopsy is often needed to differentiate benign from malignant deposits.

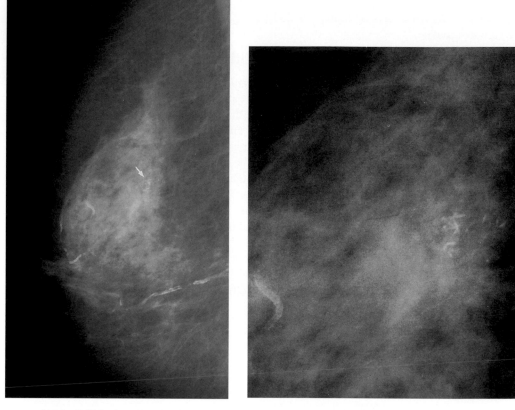

C-58. DCIS. Clustered calcifications *(A) (arrow)* are pleomorphic on closer inspection *(B)* with many irregular forms. This is highly suspicious and proved to be poorly differentiated DCIS.

Teaching Point: The more varied the particle shapes, especially when there are linear and curvilinear forms present, the more likely the lesion will prove to be poorly differentiated DCIS.

Linearly Distributed Calcifications

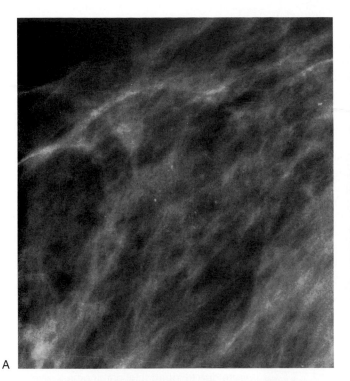

A

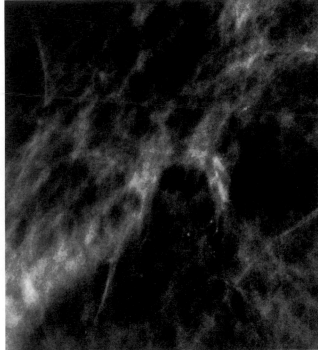

B

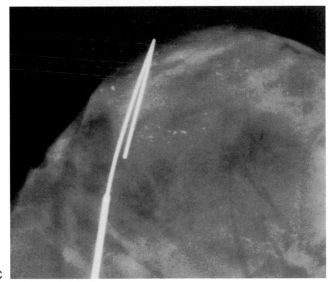

C

C-59. High-grade, poorly differentiated DCIS. These punctate calcifications that are in a linear, branching distribution, as seen on the magnification lateral *(A)* and CC *(B)* projections, were biopsied and proved to be poorly differentiated DCIS. Their small size is evident at the edge of the specimen radiograph *(C)*, which was obtained at 1.5 times magnification and has been photographically enlarged.

Teaching Point: The surgeon should be alerted when calcifications come to the margin of the specimen. This indicates that there is likely residual disease remaining in the breast.

Segmentally Distributed Calcifications

[See *Breast Imaging, Second Edition*, p. 335.]

Since intraductal cancer has a propensity to grow up and down the branches of the ducts. Calcifications that appear to be confined to a segment of the breast should raise concern. If the shapes of the particles are round and regular, then they are likely due to benign "stromal" deposits. If they are pleomorphic, then malignancy is likely.

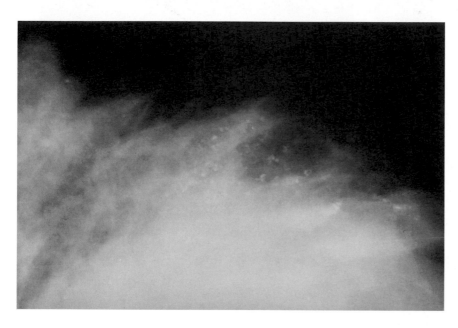

C-60. Segmentally distributed calcifications. This enlarged view of the lateral mammogram of a 33-year-old woman reveals pleomorphic calcifications that delineate a triangular, segmental distribution and were due to intraductal carcinoma.

Teaching Point: Segmentally distributed calcifications warrant careful evaluation. Unless they are very round and regular, they should be viewed with suspicion.

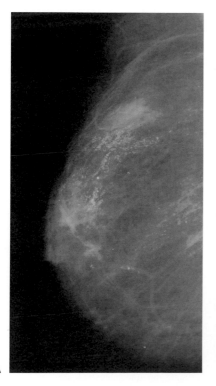

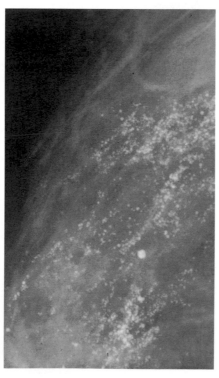

A

B

C-61. Poorly differentiated DCIS. These innumerable calcifications *(A)* are on the optically enlarged image *(B)* somewhat pleomorphic and very dense for their size. They are in a segmental distribution and were due to comedonecrosis.

Teaching Point: Segmentally distributed calcifications are suspicious.

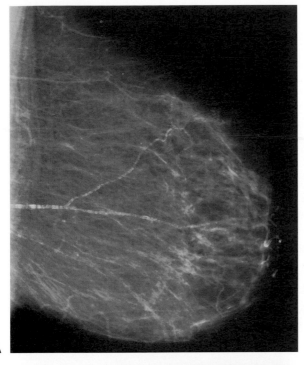

A

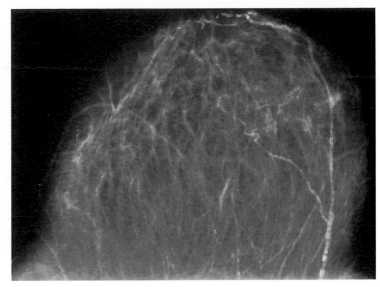

B

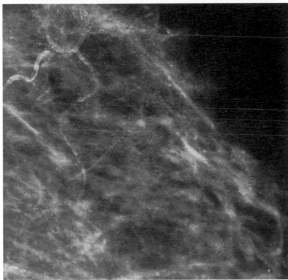

C

C-62. Punctate segmentally distributed calcifications. Very small, punctate calcifications are visible in a segmental distribution extending from the upper, outer quadrant of the right breast on the MLO *(A)* and CC *(B)* projections. Their pinpoint appearance is seen on the optically enlarged MLO *(C)*. They proved to be benign "stromal calcifications."

Teaching Point: Not all segmentally distributed calcifications are due to cancer.

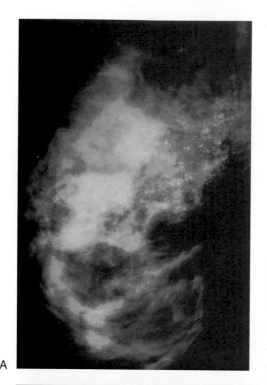

A

C-63. Segmentally distributed calcifications. These segmentally distributed calcifications on the MLO *(A)* and CC *(B)* projections are extremely pleomorphic. There is virtually no other diagnosis but DCIS. This proved to be high-grade DCIS.

Teaching Point: Note that the individual particles are extremely dense for their very small size. This is often a characteristic of malignant deposits. This, coupled with pleomorphism and segmental distribution, makes malignancy almost certain.

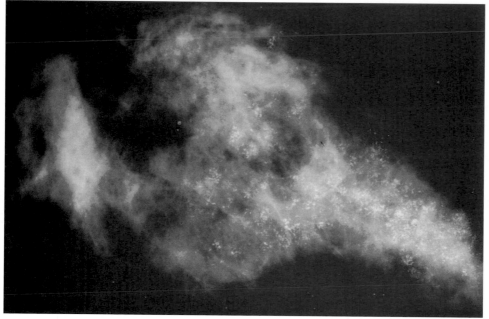

B

Regionally Distributed Calcifications

[See *Breast Imaging, Second Edition,* pp. 335–336.]

The more widespread the calcifications, the more likely they are due to a benign process. Calcifications that occupy a large volume of tissue, but not the entire breast, are termed "regionally distributed." Unfortunately, some intraductal cancers can be extremely widespread, and if the particles are pleomorphic, then cancer is likely.

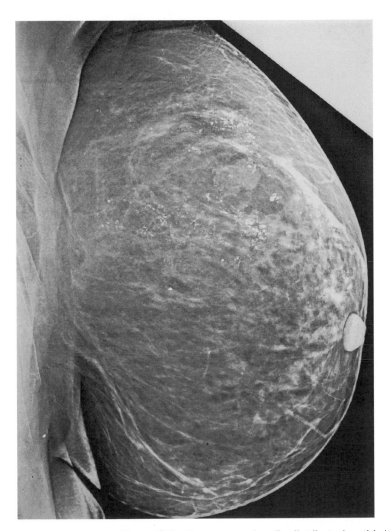

C-64. Intraductal carcinoma. The calcifications are regionally distributed on this lateral xerogram (or over a large segment), but the particles are pleomorphic in their shapes. They proved to be caused by widespread intraductal carcinoma.

Teaching Point: These are not typically benign, randomly distributed, widely scattered deposits, but rather innumerable pleomorphic deposits conforming to a large segment of the breast consistent with the diagnosis. Don't dismiss calcifications simply because they are over a fairly large region.

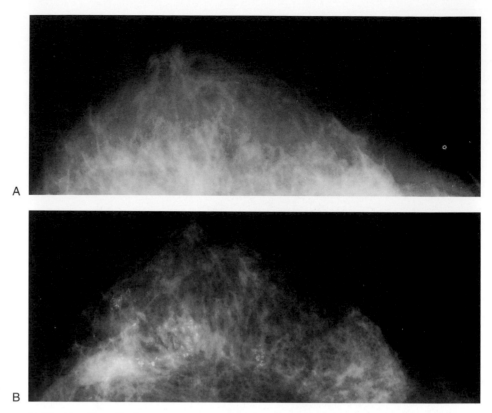

C-65. Postirradiation recurrent cancer. *(A)* This is the craniocaudal projection of a woman who had been treated with lumpectomy and radiation therapy for breast cancer. The breast is edematous from the treatment and difficult to compress *(B)*. Two years later, she has developed innumerable pleomorphic calcifications in a large region of the breast that were found to be due to recurrent breast cancer.

Teaching Point: Although benign, dystrophic calcifications are fairly common in irradiated breasts following lumpectomy. When the calcifications are small and pleomorphic, recurrence should be suspected.

Diffusely Scattered Calcifications

Diffusely scattered calcifications, particularly when bilateral, almost invariably represent a benign process. Benign forms tend to have similar shapes. This usually permits their differentiation from the more heterogeneous calcifications of diffuse breast cancer. Diffusely scattered, benign calcifications tend to be amorphous and are likely in "burned-out" lobules.

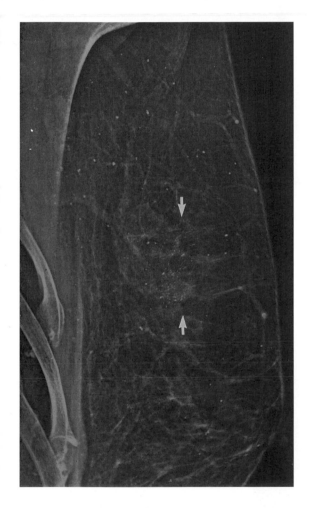

C-66. Skin calcifications. Diffusely scattered calcifications, each under 2 to 3 mm in size, with lucent centers may be found in the skin, as seen on this lateral xerogram. Note the difference between these and the large group of pleomorphic calcifications in the center *(arrows)* that proved to be ductal carcinoma *in situ.*

Teaching Point: Skin calcifications are likely when the particles are diffusely scattered. Nevertheless, avoid the "instant happiness" syndrome and keep looking even if you have found something.

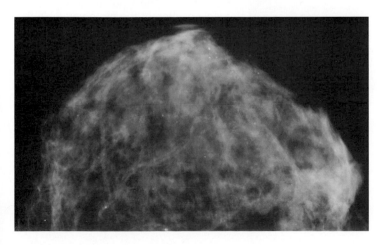

C-67. Amorphous, diffusely scattered calcifications. It has been suggested that when calcifications are spread diffusely throughout the breast, they represent "adenosis." The data for this are not clear, but, unless the particles are heterogeneous in their shapes, these calcifications are virtually always due to a benign process, and intervention is not indicated.

Teaching Point: The more you look, the more you see. Diffusely scattered calcifications should be in all parts of the breast. They are virtually always benign.

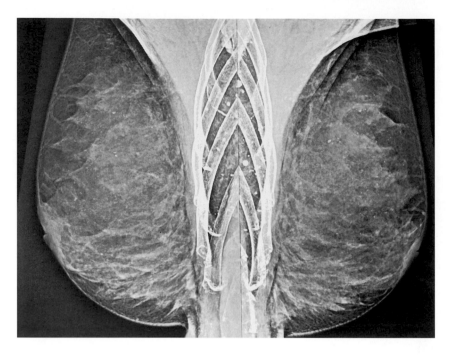

C-68. Benign, diffusely scattered calcifications. There are innumerable, amorphous, scattered calcifications in both breasts, as seen on these negative mode xeromammographic laterals. The histology that produced them is not known, but they are the result of some benign process.

Teaching Point: Calcifications that are diffuse, bilateral, and similar in their amorphous shapes are the result of benign processes.

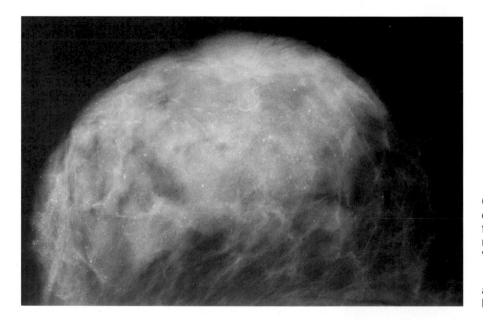

C-69. Benign, diffusely scattered calcifications. The small amorphous, diffusely scattered (the more you look, the more you see) calcifications are likely in "burned-out" lobules.

Teaching Point: Diffusely scattered, amorphous calcifications are due to a benign process.

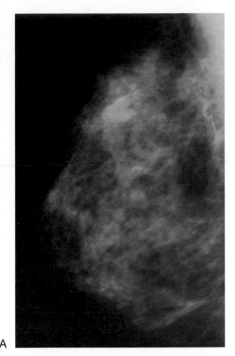
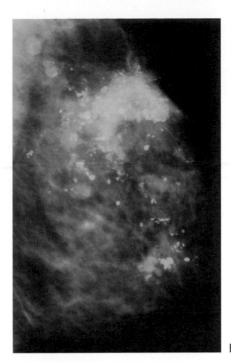

A B

C-70. Markedly asymmetric, diffusely scattered calcifications are very unusual. In this patient the left breast, as seen on the lateral mammogram *(A)*, was unremarkable. The pronounced asymmetry, pleomorphism, and exuberance of the calcifications in the right breast *(B)* led to their biopsy, revealing diffuse intraductal cancer.

Teaching Point: Diffuse intraductal cancer is very rare. If the morphology of the particles is heterogeneous, or there is a great imbalance (only on one side), as in this case, then sampling of the tissue is recommended.

Section III:
Masses and Architectural Distortion on Mammograms

[See *Breast Imaging, Second Edition*, pp. 267–315.]

ROUND AND OVAL MASSES WITH SHARPLY DEFINED MARGINS

[See *Breast Imaging, Second Edition*, pp. 279–281.]

On a statistical basis, round or oval masses with smooth, sharply circumscribed margins are almost always benign. Approximately 2% to 5% of circumscribed masses that are biopsied prove to be malignant. A lucent ring, or "halo," may appear surrounding a mass. This merely means that the macroscopic margins are distinct from the surrounding tissue, resulting in an optical illusion (the Mach effect). Although circumscribed, smooth-margined masses with halos are almost always benign, *the halo is not an absolute indication of a benign process.* Each mass should be considered individually. Margin analysis can be improved by magnification imaging. Ultrasound may help determine cystic or solid characteristics. Some have suggested that round, well-defined cancers are more indolent, but there are no good data supporting this.

Many "circumscribed" masses actually have a part of their margin obscured by overlapping or adjacent normal tissue. Sickles requires 75% of the margin to be sharply defined in two orthogonal magnification images for a lesion to be classified as being basically circumscribed with a partially obscured margin (personal communication). Based on Sickles's long-term follow-up study of these lesions, and because of the low probability of malignancy for these lesions, many practitioners feel they can be safely followed, and intervention instituted only if they undergo change.

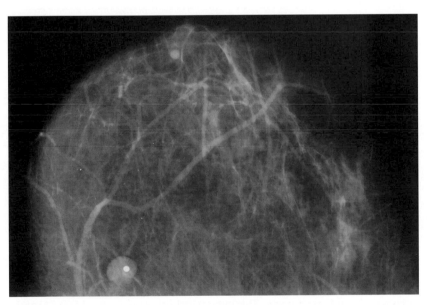

MA-1. Skin lesions may be circumscribed. This round, sharply circumscribed mass seen medially on this CC projection was a benign, epidermal inclusion cyst. The "BB" was placed on the intercutaneous mass to confirm its concordance on the mammogram.

Teaching Point: If there is a raised or hard skin lesion, the technologist should place a marker on it so that it will not raise concern on the mammogram.

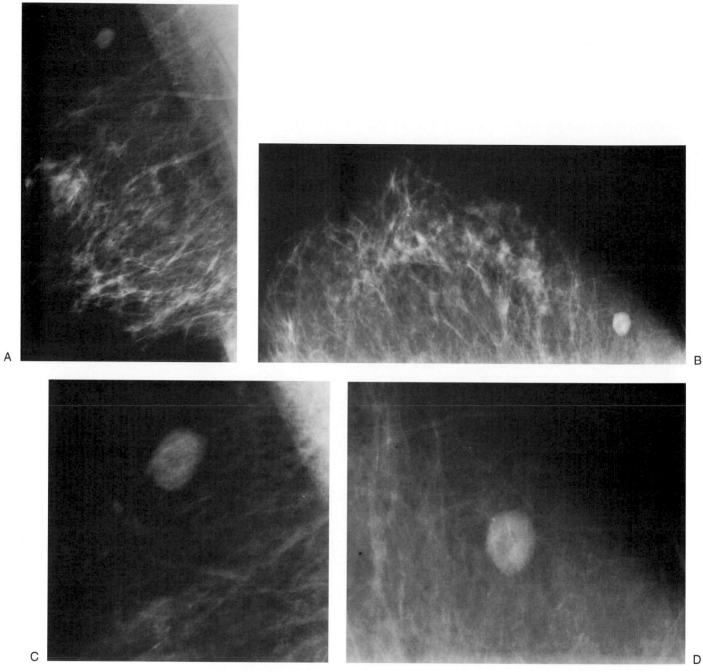

MA-2. Intramammary lymph node. This circumscribed mass on the MLO *(A)* and the CC *(B)* projections is in the typical location (upper, outer quadrant), and has the characteristic appearance, with central fat seen on the enlarged MLO *(C)* and CC *(D)* projections, of a benign intramammary lymph node.

Teaching Point: Intramammary lymph nodes are very common and are visible in 3% to 5% of mammograms. They are almost always found along the lateral edge of the breast parenchyma.

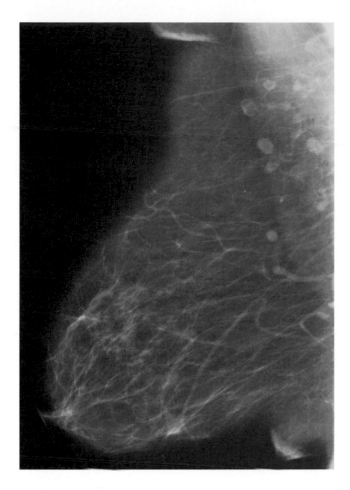

MA-3. Prepectoral lymph node. The rounded density deep in the left breast is almost certainly a prepectoral lymph node. Even though it does not clearly demonstrate a fat center, it is well defined and consistent with the diagnosis. It was unchanged over 3 years.

Teaching Point: Lymph nodes can be found deep in the breast, close to the pectoralis muscle.

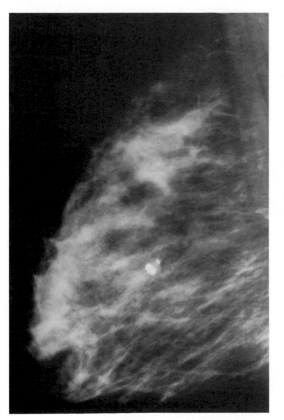

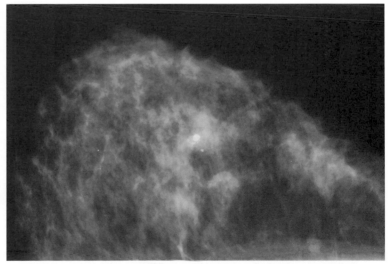

B

A

MA-4. Prepectoral lymph node. The round, circumscribed density deep in the left breast, seen on the MLO *(A)* and CC *(B)* projections was unchanged over 7 years and is almost certainly a prepectoral lymph node. A small fat center is suggested.

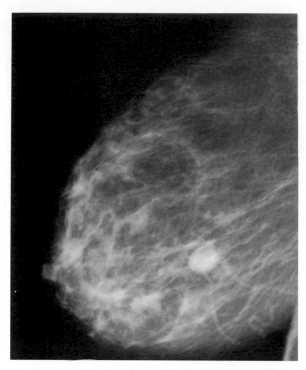

MA-5. Cyst. This solitary circumscribed mass was aspirated and confirmed to be a cyst.

Teaching Point: Most cysts are round or oval and sharply defined.

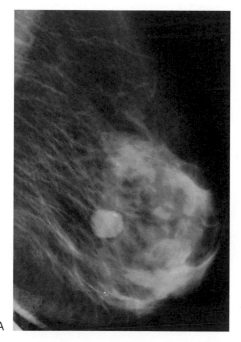

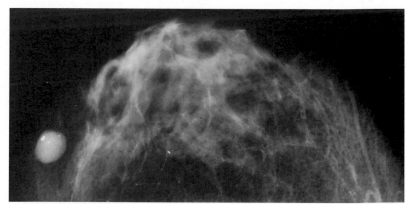

MA-6. Fibroadenoma. This sharply marginated mass on the MLO *(A)* and CC *(B)* projections in the lateral left breast has a few peripheral calcifications strongly suggestive of an involuting fibroadenoma.

Teaching Point: If a mass is round, oval, or slightly lobulated with a circumscribed margin and contains coarse, large calcifications, the diagnosis of an involuting fibroadenoma is almost certain.

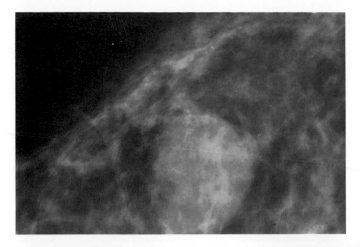

MA-7. Fibroadenoma. The palpable mass in the lateral right breast, seen on this spot compression view, was solid on ultrasound, excised, and proved to be a fibroadenoma.

Teaching Point: Although the diagnosis can be suggested, it is impossible to differentiate this fibroadenoma from a cyst, or even a circumscribed cancer by mammography. On a statistical basis it is a benign lesion, but tissue analysis is the only way to establish a certain diagnosis.

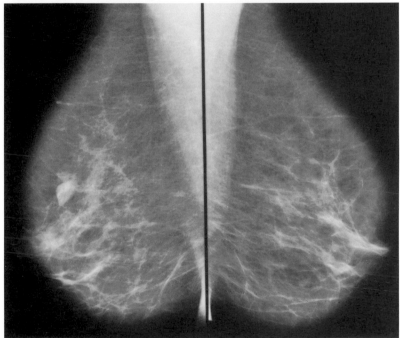

A

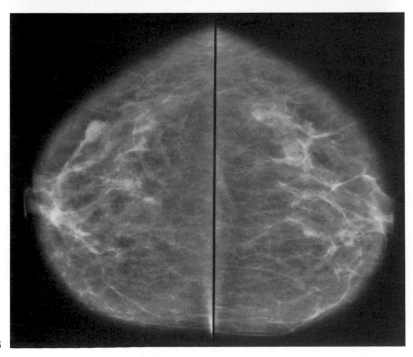

B

MA-8. Probable fibroadenoma. The circumscribed mass in the anterior *(A)* and lateral *(B)* aspect of the left breast has been unchanged for 10 years.

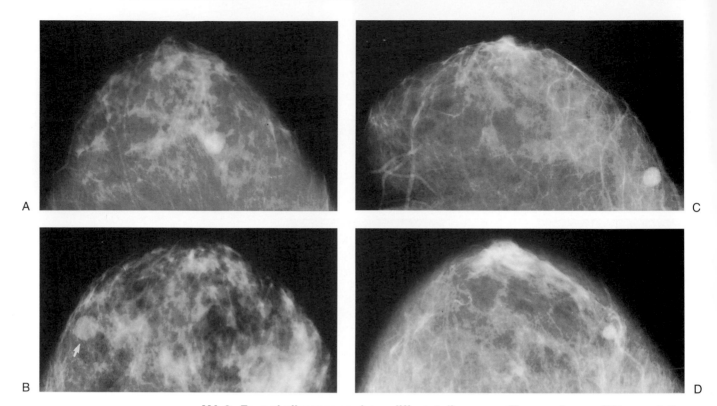

MA-9. Four similar masses have different diagnoses. The round mass *(A)* is a cyst, the second mass *(B)* proved to be a fibroadenoma, the third mass *(C)* proved to be a benign hyperplastic lymph node, and the fourth mass *(D)* was lymphoma.

Teaching Point: Different lesions may have the same appearance on mammograms.

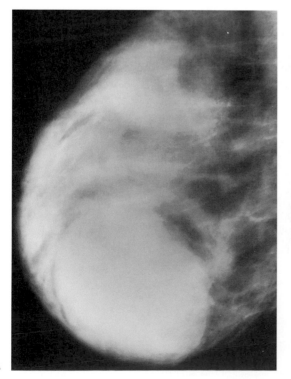

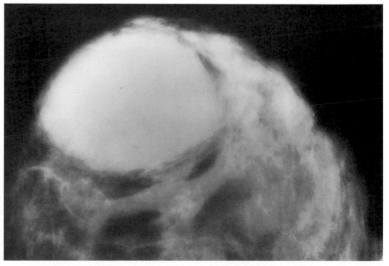

MA-10. Breast abscess. The MLO *(A)* and CC *(B)* images demonstrate a 7-cm sharply marginated mass displacing normal breast tissue in this immunosuppressed renal transplant patient. Aspiration of purulent material confirmed a staphylococcal abscess.

Teaching Point: There is nothing that distinguishes this lesion from other circumscribed masses. The history of immunosuppression suggests the possibility of an abscess.

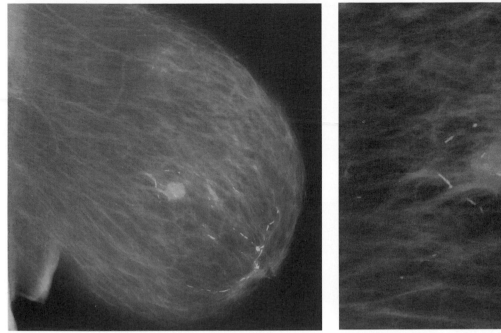
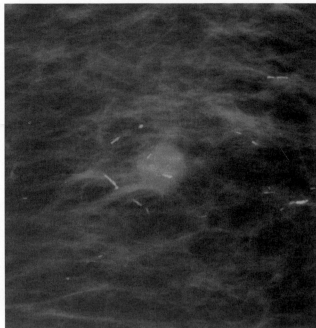

A

B

MA-11. Circumscribed cancer. *(A)* The sharply marginated mass with what appears to be a partially obscured portion on the enlarged image *(B)* proved to be invasive ductal carcinoma. The calcifications are benign secretory deposits.

Teaching Point: Breast cancer can be well defined and indistinguishable from benign lesions.

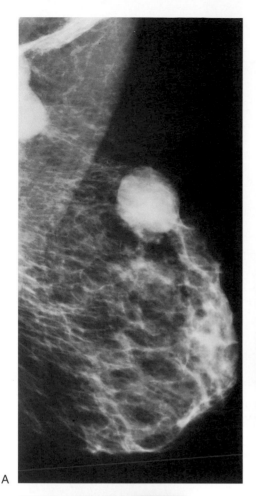

A

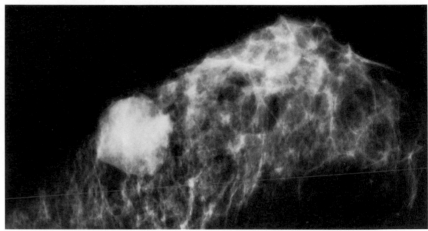

B

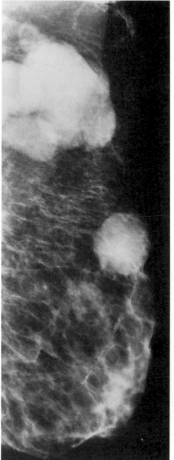

C

MA-12. Round cancer. The round mass on the MLO *(A)* and CC *(B)* proved to be a grade II invasive ductal carcinoma. On the axillary tail view *(C)* the large (21/23) positive axillary lymph nodes are evident.

Teaching Point: Circumscribed cancers are not innocuous as some have suggested. Most prove to be invasive ductal carcinoma not otherwise specified (NOS).

LOBULATED MASSES

[See *Breast Imaging, Second Edition*, pp. 281–293.]

Lobulated masses with sharply defined margins are also usually benign, but lobulations should increase the level of concern. Unfortunately, as with many characteristics of breast lesions, there is a significant overlap between benign and malignant lobulated lesions. In general, the smaller and more frequent the lobulations (see Microlobulated Masses, p. 79) the greater the concern.

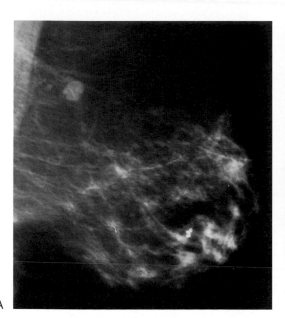
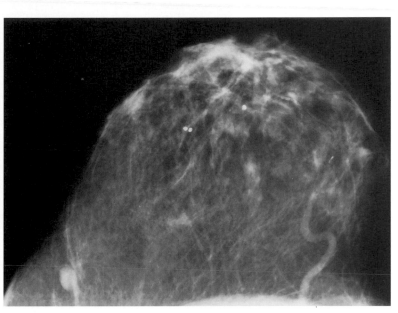

A · B

MA-13. Benign intramammary lymph node. The lobulated mass in the upper *(A)*, outer *(B)* quadrant is typical in size, shape, and location of a benign intramammary lymph node.

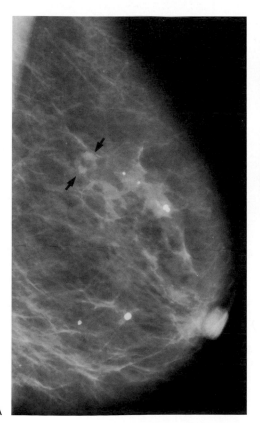
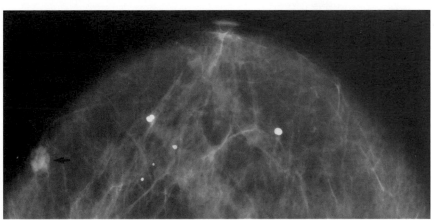

B

A

MA-14. Benign intramammary lymph node. This very lobulated, fat-containing mass in the upper *(A)* lateral *(B)* right breast has the typical appearance of a benign intramammary lymph node.

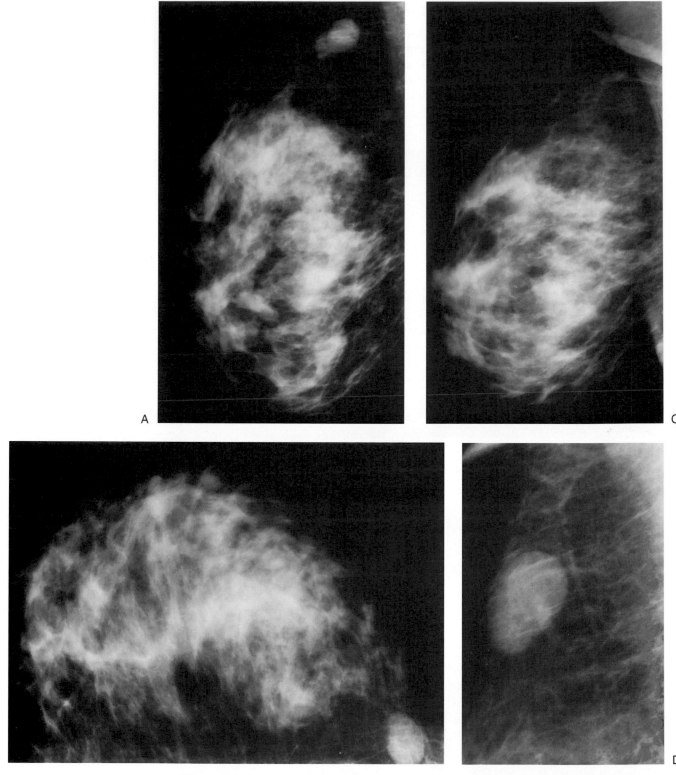

MA-15. Benign hyperplastic intramammary lymph node. The lobulated mass in the upper left breast on the lateral *(A)* and CC *(B)* projections had enlarged dramatically from the previous study *(C)*. It has a sharply defined lobulated contour on magnification *(D)* and proved to be a benign hyperplastic lymph node.

Teaching Point: Intramammary lymph nodes are frequently extremely lobulated when they contain a large amount of fat.

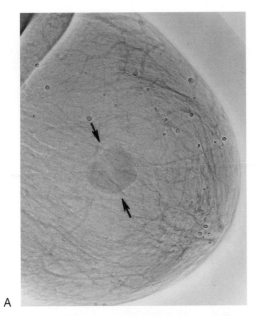

A

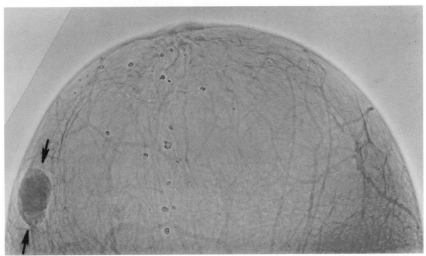

B

MA-16. Dermatopathic lymph node. The mass seen on the lateral xeromammogram *(A)* and laterally on the craniocaudal xerogram *(B)* proved to be a benign, dermatopathic lymph node.

Teaching Point: Dermatologic conditions can cause enlargement of intramammary lymph nodes. A dermatopathic node is characteristic of psoriasis.

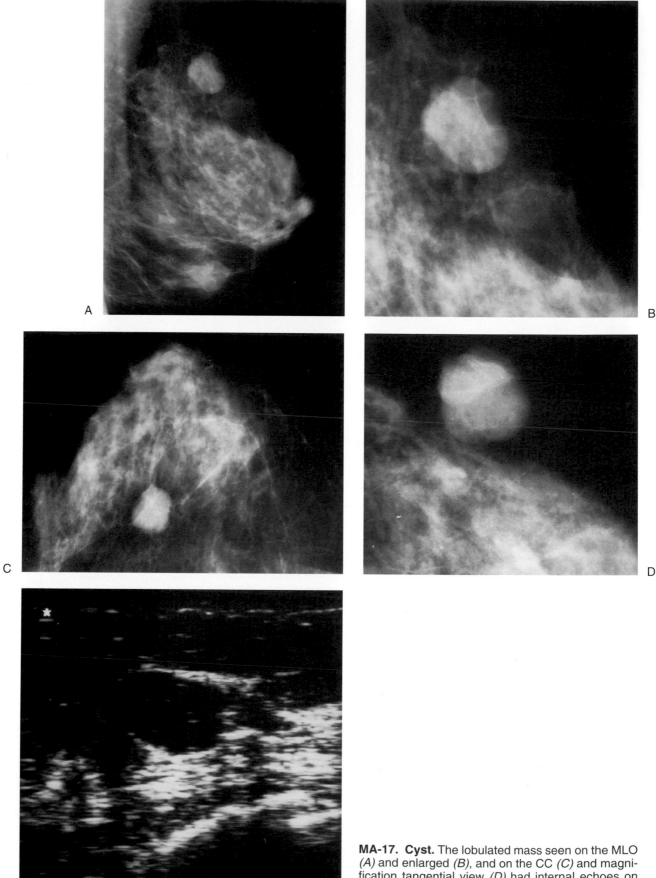

MA-17. Cyst. The lobulated mass seen on the MLO *(A)* and enlarged *(B)*, and on the CC *(C)* and magnification tangential view *(D)* had internal echoes on ultrasound *(E)*. Consequently, it was aspirated, confirming a benign, simple cyst.

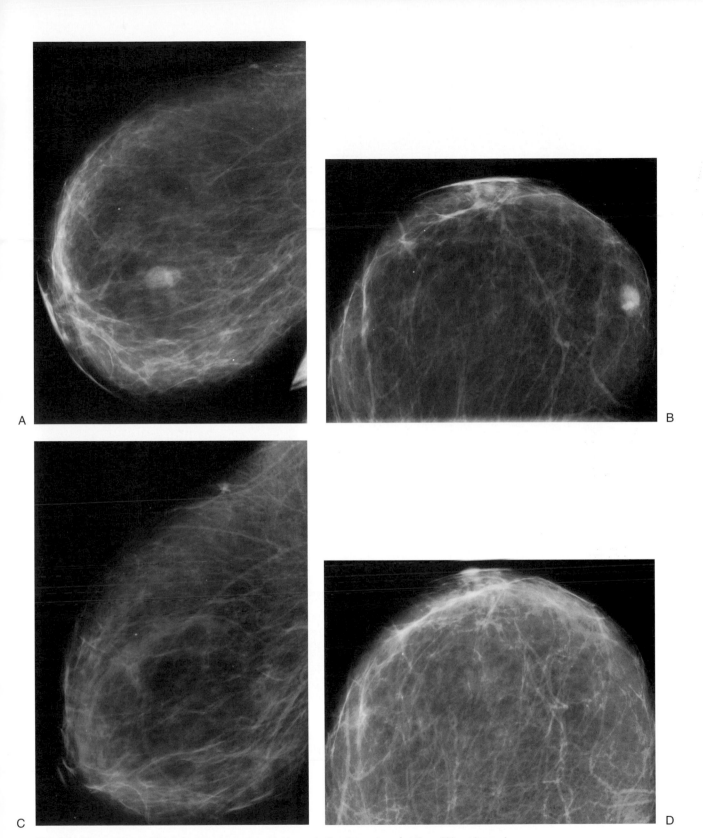

MA-18. Hematoma. The lobulated mass seen here in the lateral projection *(A)* and cranio-caudal *(B)* views occurred following trauma. The lesion was a hematoma. Several months later, repeat mammography *(C,D)* revealed complete resolution of the lesion.

Teaching Point: In the past, breast cancer was thought to be related to trauma because some cancers were detected following trauma. After sustaining an injury to the breast, the patient would notice a mass that was not a hematoma, but was actually cancer. The cancer had likely been present much earlier, but, either as a result of denial, or having not examined herself prior to the trauma, the patient was not aware of the mass. In fact, a true hematoma (blood-filled posttraumatic mass), is unusual in the breast and a lump discovered following trauma should be carefully evaluated. Nevertheless, where there is evidence of substantial trauma, as in this case, it is reasonable to follow a lesion and not intervene.

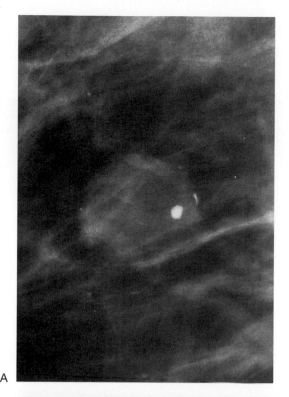

A

B

MA-19. Fibroadenoma. This lobulated mass on the magnification lateral *(A)* and the craniocaudal *(B)* projections has associated coarse calcifications that make the diagnosis almost certain.

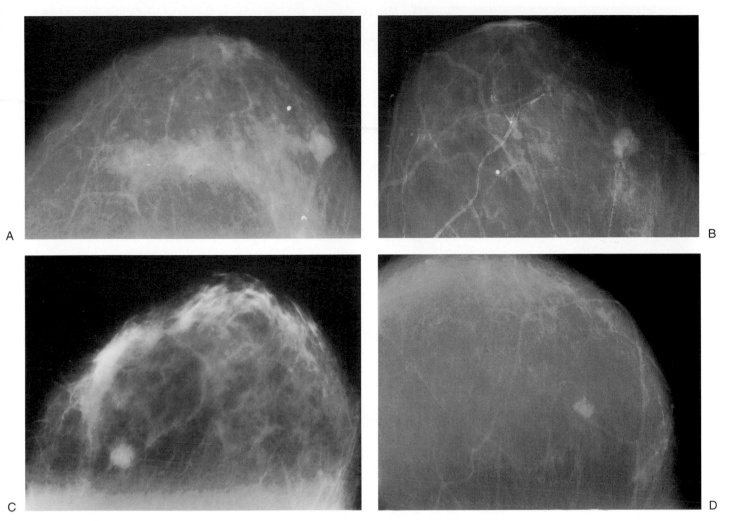

MA-20. Four similar masses with different diagnoses. The lobulated mass in the lateral left breast *(A)* proved to be a cyst. In a second patient the mass in the lateral left breast proved to be invasive ductal carcinoma *(B)*. The mass in the lateral right breast of a third patient was also invasive ductal carcinoma *(C)*. The fourth mass *(D)* proved to be an unusual hemangioma.

Teaching Point: The morphology of benign and malignant masses may overlap. Lesions with lobulated shapes should be carefully evaluated.

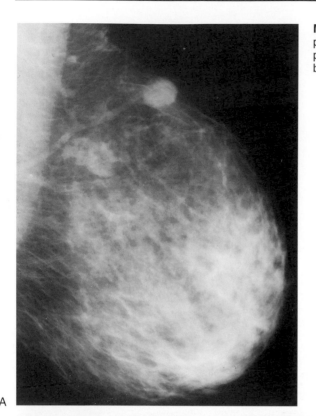

A

MA-21. Cancer. *(A)* This mass in the upper *(B)* central right breast appears fairly well defined, even on the photographic enlargement *(C)*. It proved to represent an unusual adenosquamous carcinoma of the breast.

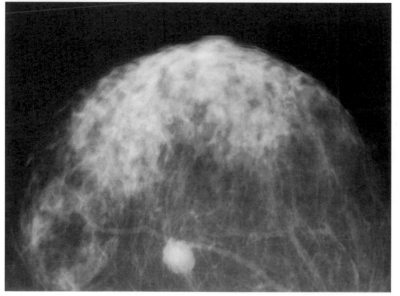

B

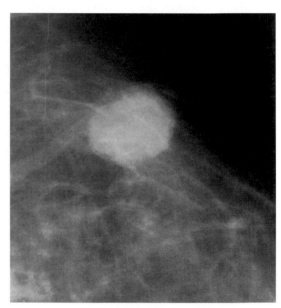

C

MICROLOBULATED MASSES

[See *Breast Imaging, Second Edition*, p. 295.]

When the lobulations are small and frequent, they are termed microlobulations. This is a fairly uncommon finding, but, when present, the likelihood of malignancy is increased.

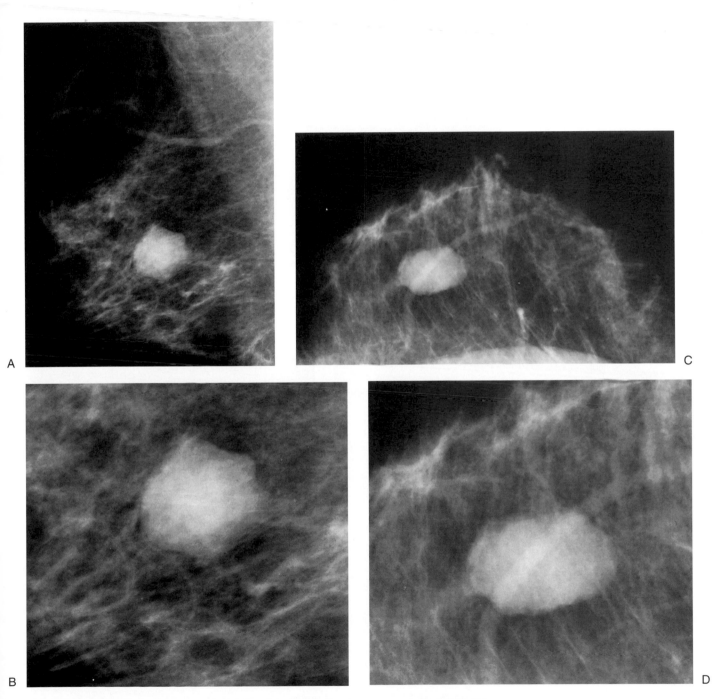

MA-22. Benign cyst. This mass with microlobulated margins seen on the MLO *(A)*, enlarged *(B)*, and CC *(C)*, enlarged *(D)*, projections proved to be a benign cyst.

Teaching Point: Since a cyst is usually due to the dilatation of the lobule and its acini, it is not surprising that it might have a microlobulated margin.

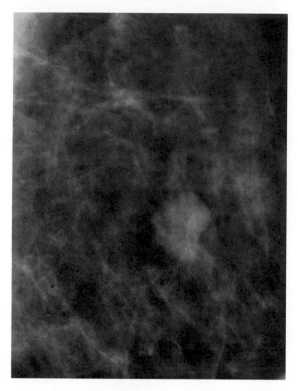

MA-23. Another microlobulated cyst. Only aspiration could prove that this was a simple cyst.

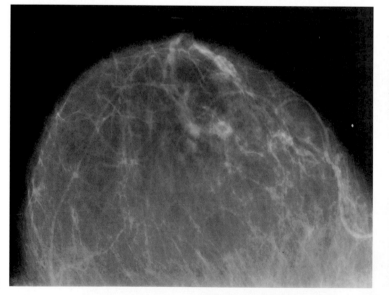
A

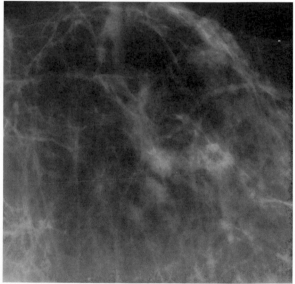
B

MA-24. Ductal carcinoma *in situ* (DCIS). This microlobulated mass seen on the CC *(A)* projection, enlarged *(B)* and on magnification lateral *(C)* mammogram, proved to be ductal carcinoma *in situ* that was expanding the duct, forming a microlobulated mass.

Teaching Point: DCIS can form a mass.

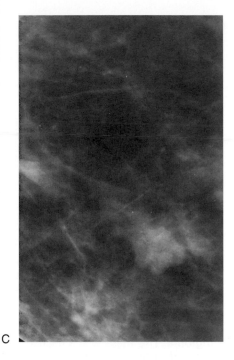

C

MA-24. *Continued*

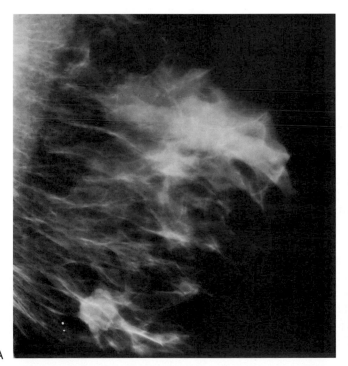

A

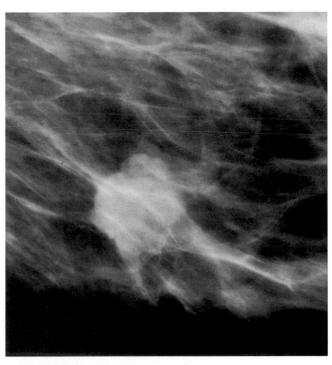

B

MA-25. Invasive ductal carcinoma. This 1.6-cm invasive ductal carcinoma is a typical cancer with a microlobulated margin seen on the MLO *(A)* and enlarged view *(B)*. It was poorly differentiated with metastatic disease found in an intramammary lymph node, although 12 axillary nodes were uninvolved.

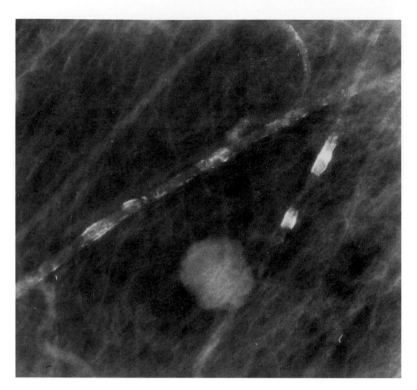

MA-26. Hemangioma. This mass with a microlobulated margin proved to be a cavernous hemangioma.

ROUND, OVAL, AND LOBULATED MASSES WITH OBSCURED MARGINS

[See *Breast Imaging, Second Edition*, p. 294.]

These are lesions that are mostly benign, which, if they were examined outside the breast, would have sharply defined margins; however, adjacent or superimposed breast tissue obscures their margin. One of the most difficult interpretive tasks is to determine whether or not a margin is ill-defined, or merely sharply defined but obscured by superimposed breast tissue. This can sometimes be determined through the use of additional projections and spot compression. Most cancers, even those that appear to be well defined, on close inspection have some ill-definition of their margin. Unfortunately, benign lesions can also have ill-defined margins. If a cyst, or fibroadenoma, develops in fibrous connective tissue, its borders may be ill-defined, regardless of the projection, since both the lesion and the tissue abutting it have the same x-ray attenuation. Ultrasound is the fastest way to determine if the lesion represents a cyst. If it is solid, a biopsy is the most accurate method of determining its etiology.

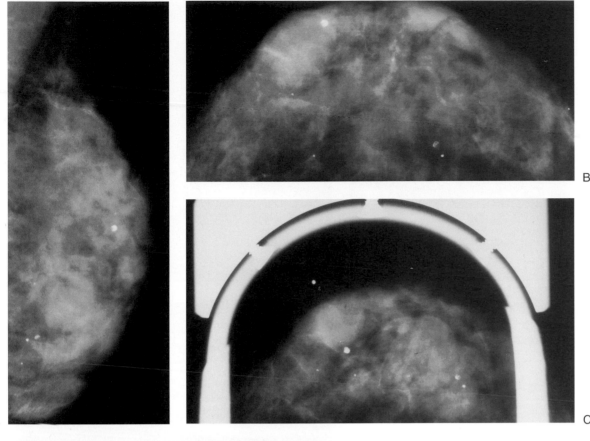

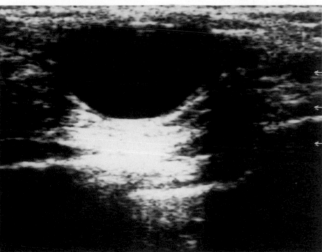

MA-27. Cyst. The palpable, ovoid mass in a 74-year-old woman is barely visible in the MLO *(A)* projection and it is obscured on the CC *(B)* projection. Spot compression *(C)* does not add to the evaluation, but ultrasound *(D)* clearly proves that the mass is a cyst and no further evaluation is needed.

Teaching Point: Postmenopausal women can have dense breast tissue and cysts. Ultrasound is the fastest way to determine whether a lesion is cystic or solid.

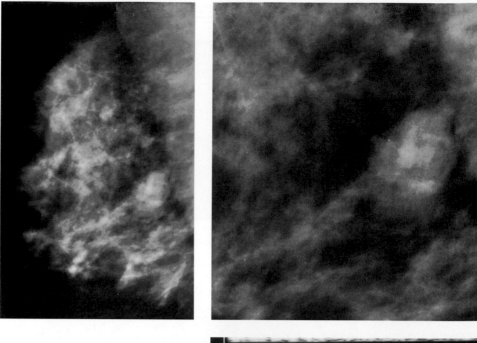

A

B

C

MA-28. Cyst. This mass was found by mammography in a 46-year-old as seen on this MLO projection *(A).* Close inspection *(B)* reveals an ovoid mass that is low in x-ray attenuation with probably obscured margins. Ultrasound *(C)* demonstrates a benign cyst.

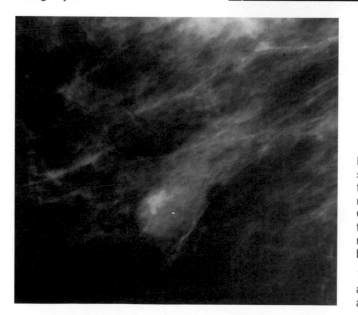

M-29. Fibroadenoma. This mass, seen on this magnification image in the lateral projection, was found by mammography in a 42-year-old. Ovoid, relatively low in x-ray attenuation, and with an obscured posterior margin, it proved by biopsy to be a fibroadenoma.

Teaching Point: Fibroadenomas and cysts can have identical appearances by mammography.

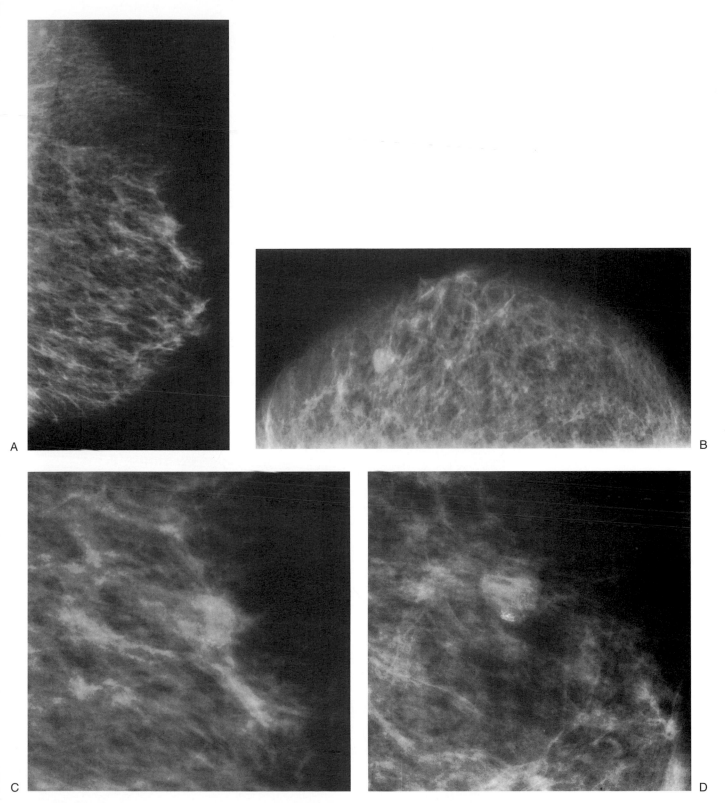

MA-30. Cancer. This round mass found by mammography anteriorly on the MLO *(A)* and laterally on the CC *(B)* projection of the right breast, is low in x-ray attenuation. Its margins are obscured as seen on the enlarged MLO *(C)*, and magnification lateral *(D)*. Biopsy revealed a papillary carcinoma with associated cribriform (low grade) DCIS (note the punctate calcifications on *C* and *D*).

Teaching Point: In the analysis of a specific lesion it is frequently not possible to differentiate benign masses from malignant without a biopsy.

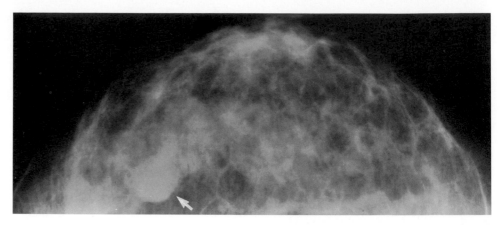

MA-31. Cyst. This circumscribed mass with an obscured margin in the lateral right breast on the CC projection is quite dense, but proved to be a benign, simple cyst.

Teaching Point: Cysts can have fairly high attenuation. They should completely resolve with aspiration.

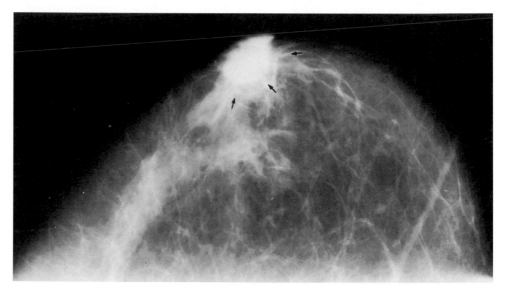

MA-32. Cancer. The high attenuation mass in the subareolar region of the right breast *(arrows)* on this craniocaudal projection is an ovoid mass with an obscured margin. It proved to be invasive ductal carcinoma.

Teaching Point: Breast cancer is usually fairly high in x-ray attenuation.

IRREGULARLY SHAPED MASSES WITH ILL-DEFINED MARGINS

[See *Breast Imaging, Second Edition*, pp. 295–298.]

The more irregular the shape and ill-defined the margin of a mass, the greater the likelihood of malignancy. Ill-defined masses can be extremely hard to evaluate and are frequently only islands of normal breast tissue. Before suggesting the possibility of a malignancy, one must determine that a lesion is in fact real. This can be accomplished by varying the projection and compression. Another difficult distinction is differentiating an ill-defined margin from a sharply defined lesion whose margin is obscured by overlying normal tissue. As noted above, many circumscribed masses actually have a part of their margin obscured. Sickles requires 75% of the margin to be sharply defined in two orthogonal magnification images for a lesion to be classified as being basically circumscribed with a partially obscured margin.

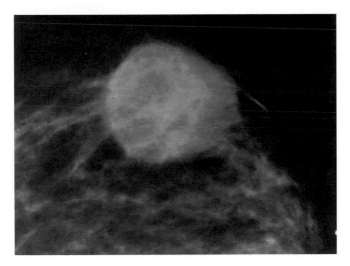

MA-33. Hematoma. This rounded mass with an ill-defined margin was a hematoma that formed 7 days following the excision of an invasive breast cancer. It eventually resolved.

Teaching Point: If a mass is surrounded by fat, its indistinct margins are due to the fact that it is not circumscribed.

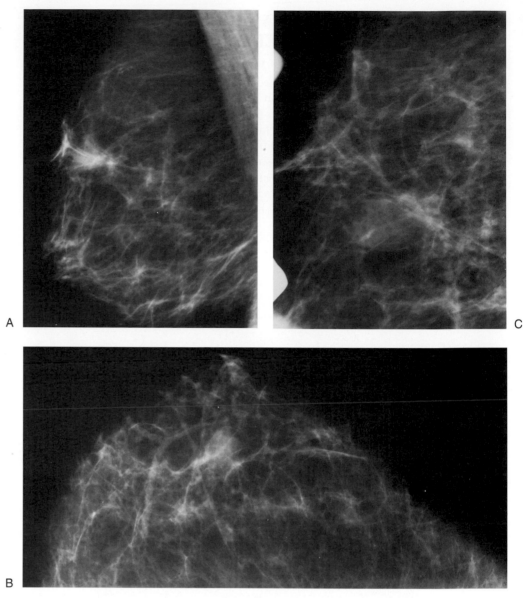

MA-34. The ill-defined mass in the upper left breast on the MLO *(A)*, and the anterior central portion on the CC *(B)* remains ill-defined on the spot compression magnification view in the lateral projection *(C)*. It proved to be a fibroadenoma.

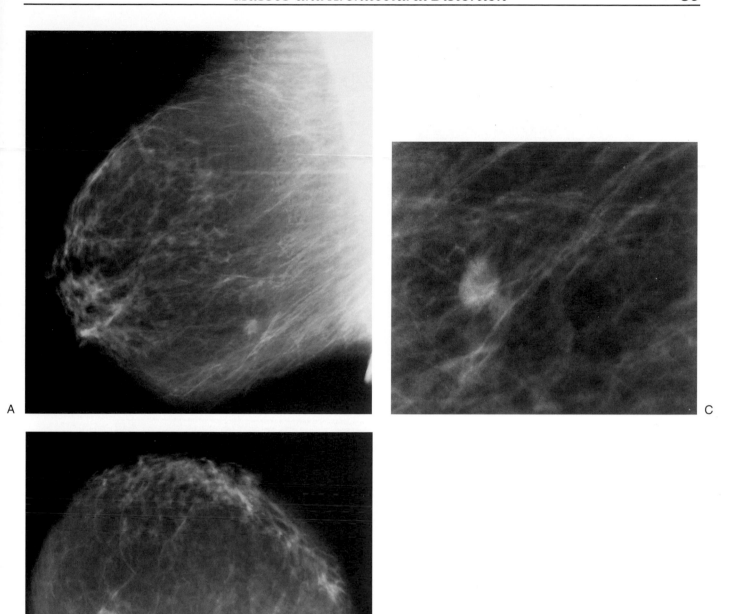

MA-35. Focal fibrosis. This ovoid mass with an ill-defined margin on the MLO *(A)* and CC *(B)* projections and on the magnification lateral *(C)* was excised and found to be benign focal fibrosis.

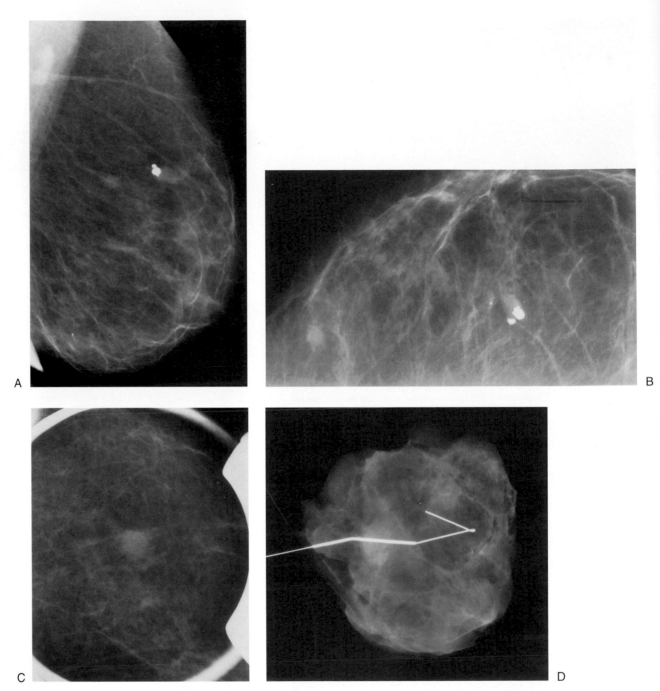

MA-36. Breast cancer. The irregular mass that is low in x-ray attenuation on the MLO *(A)* and CC *(B)* projections in the upper outer right breast is very low in x-ray attenuation. It remains ill-defined on spot compression *(C)* and on the specimen radiograph *(D)*. Biopsy revealed infiltrating ductal carcinoma. The calcifying mass anterior and more central is a benign, involuting fibroadenoma.

Teaching Point: Invasive breast cancer can be low in x-ray attenuation.

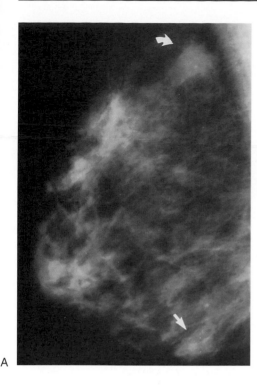

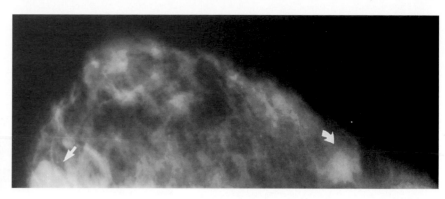

A

B

MA-37. Breast cancer and a fibroadenoma. The irregular, ill-defined lesion in the upper *(A)* outer *(B)* quadrant *(curved arrow)* proved to be an invasive ductal carcinoma, while the irregular lesion with an ill-defined margin in the lower inner quadrant *(straight arrow)* was a benign fibroadenoma.

Teaching Point: Sometimes you just can't tell.

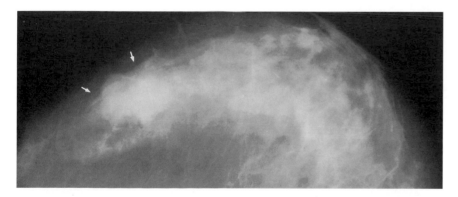

MA-38. Adenoid cystic carcinoma. The irregular mass with an ill-defined margin *(arrows)* in the lateral right breast proved to be an unusual adenoid cystic carcinoma.

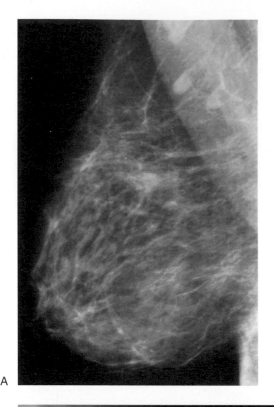

A

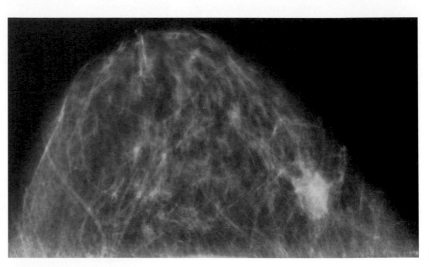

B

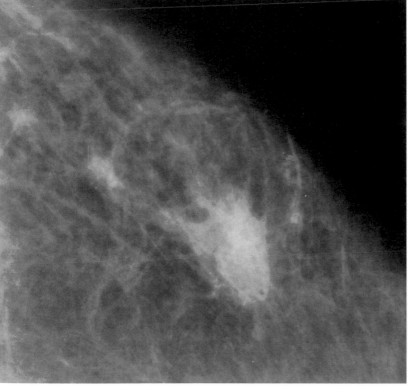

C

MA-39. Invasive ductal carcinoma. This mass has an irregular shape, with an ill-defined margin as seen on the MLO *(A)* and CC *(B)* projections as well as on the enlarged CC *(C)*. Biopsy revealed an invasive ductal carcinoma with a moderate intraductal component.

Teaching Point: Screening should involve two views. The lesion is low in attenuation and barely visible on the MLO, but it is obvious on the CC.

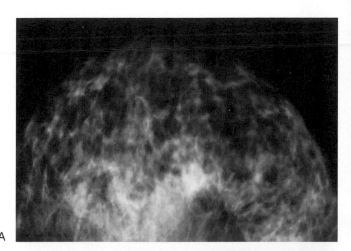

A

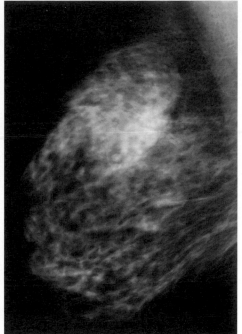

B

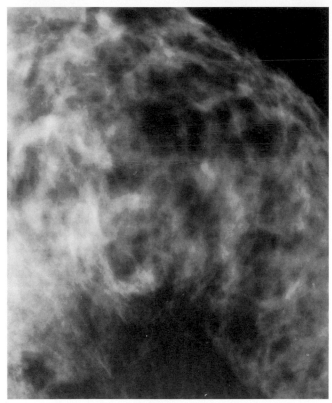

C

MA-40. Superimposed normal tissues. There appears to be an ill-defined, dense area on the CC projection *(A)* that is not visible on the MLO *(B)*. A spot compression view *(C)* in the CC projection fails to confirm an abnormality.

Teaching Point: Normal tissue can superimpose and appear to be a lesion. If there is no corroborating abnormality in the other projection, return to the view on which you see it and modify that projection to confirm that it is real.

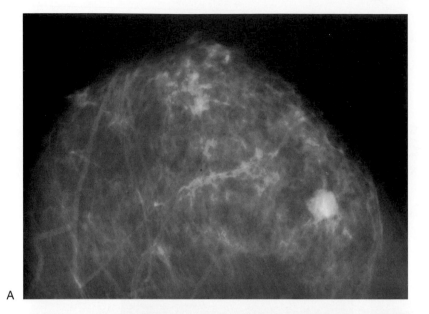

A

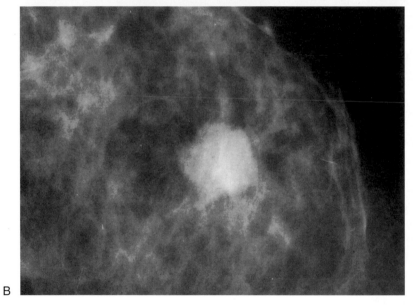

B

MA-41. Invasive breast cancer. This is a lobulated mass *(A)* that, on close inspection *(B)*, has an
ill-defined margin and proved to be invasive ductal
carcinoma.

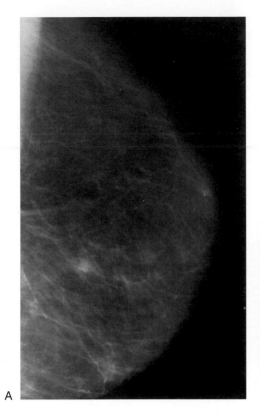

A

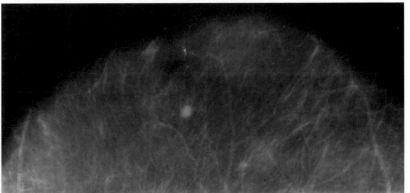

B

MA-42. Invasive breast cancer. The ill-defined mass in the right breast in the lateral *(A)*, CC *(B)*, and enlarged CC *(C)* projections is very dense for its size and proved to be an invasive ductal carcinoma.

Teaching Point: Cancer frequently forms a mass that is very dense for its size.

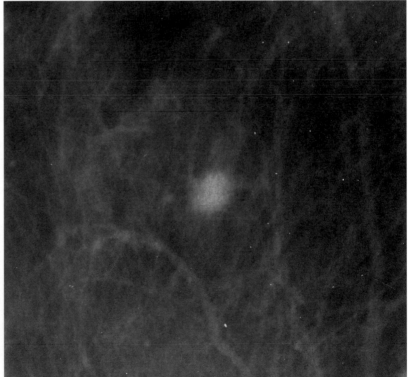

C

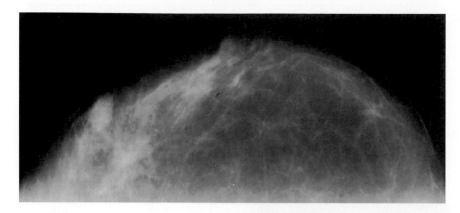

MA-43. Metastatic disease to an intra-mammary lymph node. The ill-defined mass in the outer right breast on this cranio-caudal projection proved to be an intra-mammary lymph node that was involved with tumor from the adjacent primary breast cancer.

Teaching Point: Not all upper outer quadrant masses are benign intramammary lymph nodes. Shapes and margin characteristics are important. Metastatic disease to an intramammary lymph node carries the same prognostic significance as metastatic disease to axillary lymph nodes.

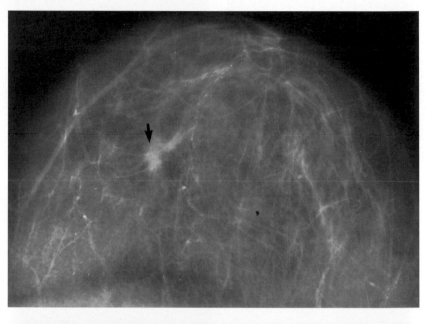

A

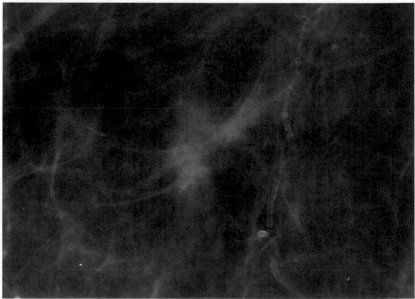

B

MA-44. Cancer. The irregular, ill-defined mass *(arrow)* in the center of the right breast *(A)* and enlarged *(B)* is not very dense for its size. Nevertheless, it proved to be an invasive ductal carcinoma. What appear to be spicules are actually, coincidental, normal Cooper's ligaments.

Teaching Point: Breast cancer is not always dense for its diameter.

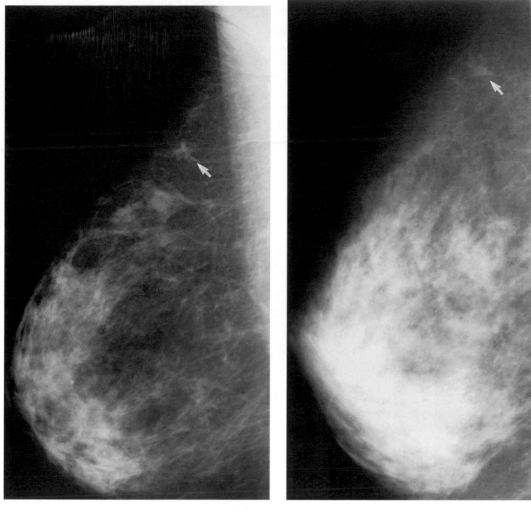

A   B

MA-45. Cancer and benign fibrosis. The irregular, ill-defined mass *(arrow) (A)*, in this patient, proved to be a small, invasive breast cancer. A very similar finding *(arrow)* in this second patient *(B)* proved to be benign fibrosis.

Teaching Point: Sometimes you just can't tell.

SPICULATED LESIONS

[See *Breast Imaging, Second Edition*, pp. 302–305.]

Virtually all spiculated lesions that are not due to previous surgery are malignant. There are a few benign lesions that are spiculated. Postsurgical spiculation usually clears over time if the excised lesion had been benign. Benign elastotic lesions of the breast (radial scars) also produce spiculation, but they usually produce distorted architecture without a mass (see Architectural Distortion, below). Granular cell tumors and extraabdominal desmoids are spiculated masses, but are extremely rare.

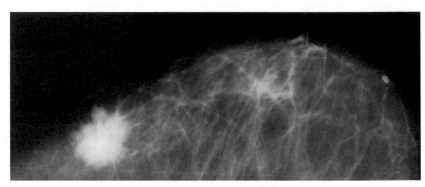

B

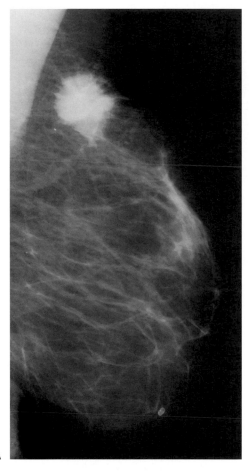

A

MA-46. Spiculated breast cancer. This infiltrating ductal carcinoma was palpable. It has the typical appearance of an irregular mass with a spiculated margin on the MLO *(A)* and CC exaggerated laterally *(B)* projections.

Teaching Point: By the time a cancer is this large, mammography has little benefit. Mammography's value is in finding earlier stage cancers.

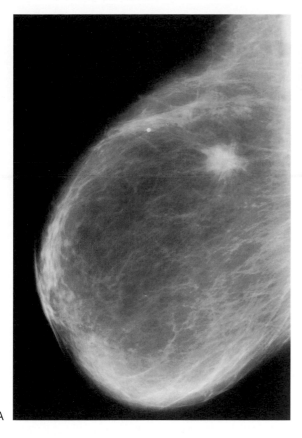

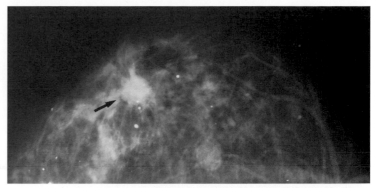

A

B

MA-47. Spiculated cancer. This large irregular mass, which proved to be invasive ductal carcinoma *(A)*, has long spicules. This smaller mass *(arrow)*, in a second patient, also has long spicules *(B)*.

Teaching Point: The size of the cancer is measured by the diameter of the mass. The length of the spicules has no apparent significance.

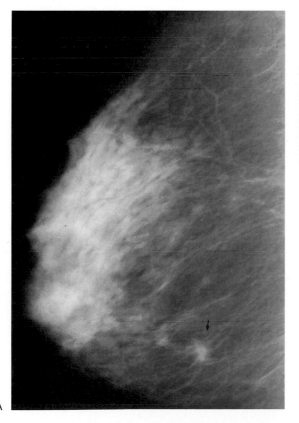

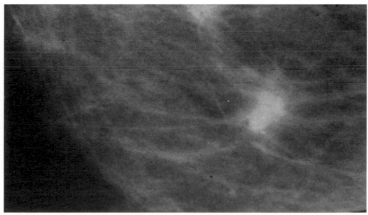

A

B

MA-48. Small, occult invasive breast cancer. The irregular, spiculated mass *(arrow) (A)* and enlarged *(B)* is a clinically occult, invasive breast cancer detected by mammography.

Teaching Point: Mammography's greatest value lies in the detection of small, early-stage breast cancers before they become clinically evident.

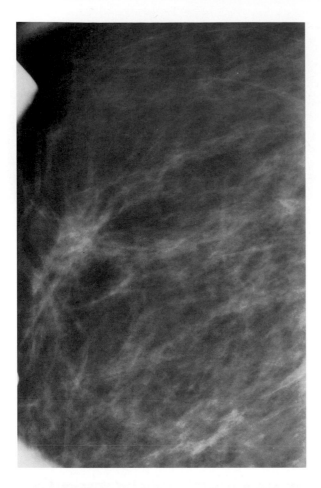

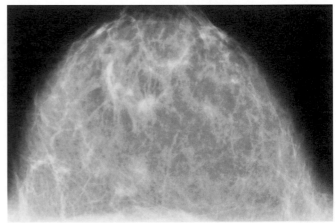

MA-49. Occult invasive breast cancer. The subtle spiculated lesion seen with magnification at the front of the breast was an early invasive breast cancer.

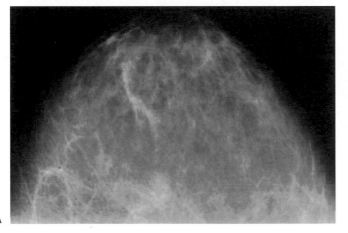

A   B

MA-50. Development of a spiculated cancer. No abnormality is evident on this cranio-caudal projection *(A)*. Two years later a small, 9-mm spiculated mass has developed in the anterior central portion of the breast *(B)*. Biopsy confirmed an invasive ductal carcinoma.

Teaching Point: The development of a spiculated mass in the absence of recent surgery virtually guarantees that the lesion is malignant. Change can be subtle.

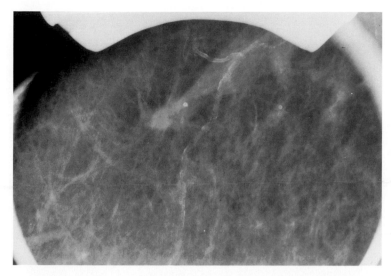

MA-51. Subtle invasive breast cancer. This looked like a vague density on the contact images. The spot compression magnification view revealed an 8-mm spiculated mass that proved to be invasive ductal carcinoma.

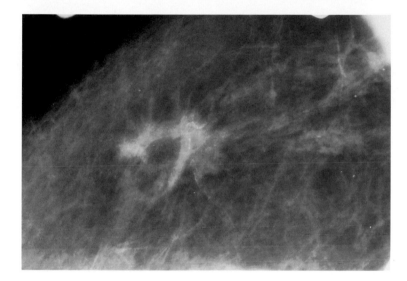

MA-52. Invasive breast cancer. This irregularly shaped mass with a spiculated margin proved to be breast cancer.

Teaching Point: Breast cancer does not always form a central mass. The fact that this lesion has trapped some fat does not make it a fat-containing lesion and does not negate its irregular shape and spiculation. A biopsy is indicated.

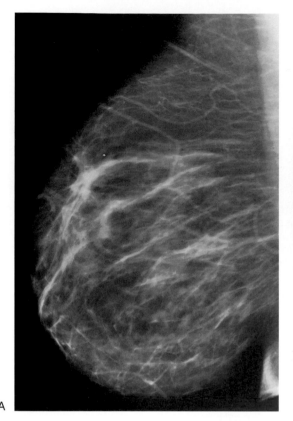

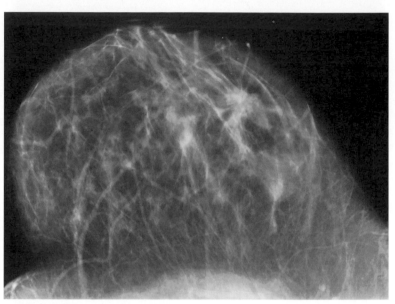

A

B

MA-53. Invasive breast cancer. The spiculated mass is difficult to see in the anterior portion of the upper left breast due to overlapping normal tissues on the MLO *(A)*. It is more easily seen on the craniocaudal projection *(B)*.

Teaching Point: Two views are needed for screening.

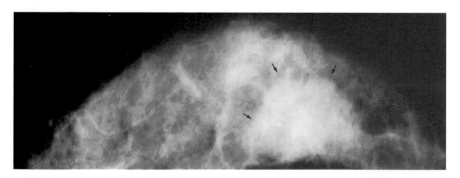

MA-54. Adenoid cystic carcinoma. This spiculated mass represents an unusual form of invasive breast cancer.

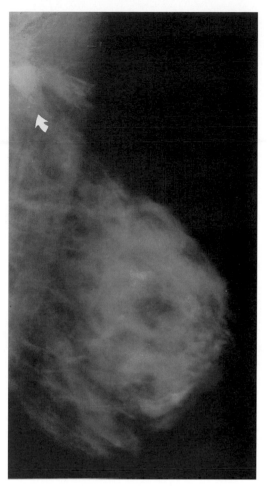

MA-55. Extraabdominal desmoid tumor. This is an example of a very rare benign extraabdominal desmoid tumor with long spicules.

Teaching Point: Based on a small series, desmoid tumors in the breast are found in close proximity to the pectoralis major muscle and have long spicules. Biopsy is still indicated since the appearance is not sufficient to exclude malignancy.

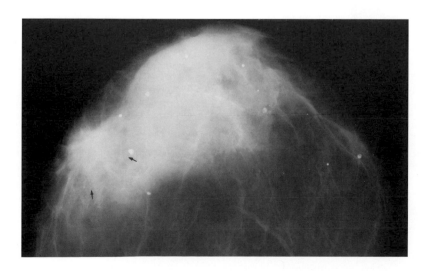

MA-56. Postsurgical change. This irregular, spiculated mass is in an area where a benign lesion had been surgically removed 4 months earlier.

Teaching Point: The breast usually heals with little evident change following a biopsy for a benign abnormality. Spiculated architectural distortion can persist for as long as 12 to 18 months, but it almost always resolves.

FOCAL ASYMMETRIC DENSITY

[See *Breast Imaging, Second Edition*, pp. 256–265.]

The breasts are generally symmetric, but focal asymmetries are common. Most asymmetries can be dismissed as normal tissues, but additional imaging may be needed to differentiate normal tissues from significant pathology.

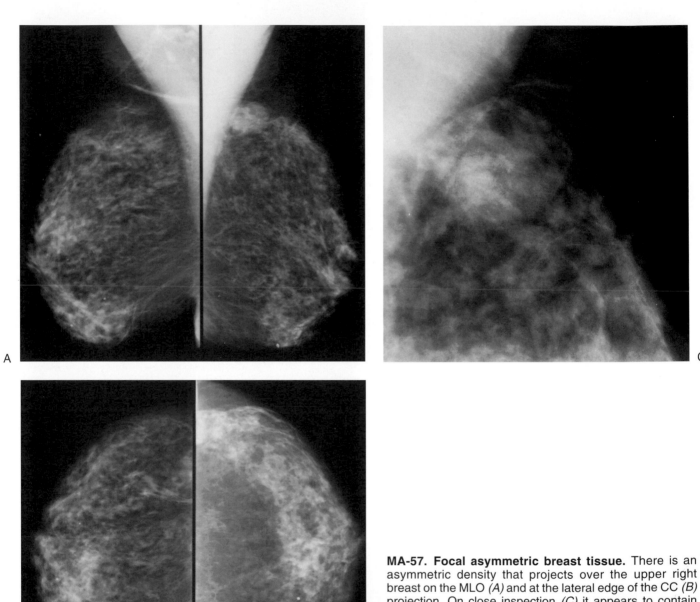

MA-57. Focal asymmetric breast tissue. There is an asymmetric density that projects over the upper right breast on the MLO *(A)* and at the lateral edge of the CC *(B)* projection. On close inspection *(C)* it appears to contain fat. It has been present for 9 years on previous mammograms and, presumably, represents focal asymmetric breast tissue. A mass that is stable for this length of time is benign.

Teaching Point: Most focal asymmetries are normal breast tissue.

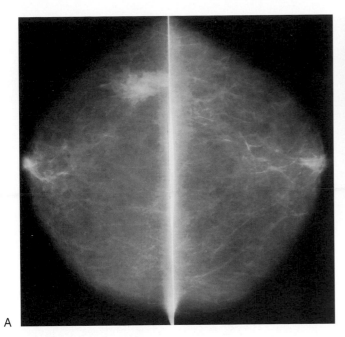

A

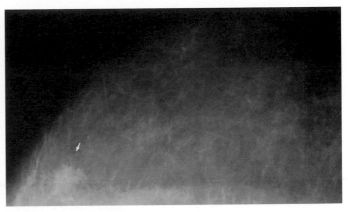

B

MA-58. Fibrosis and breast cancer. The focal asymmetry in the lateral left breast *(A)* was sufficiently irregular that it was biopsied, and proved to be benign breast tissue. It is indistinguishable from the density seen on this second case *(B)* that proved to be an invasive breast cancer.

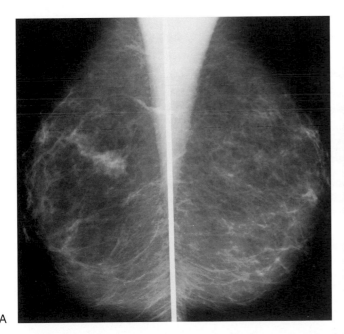

A

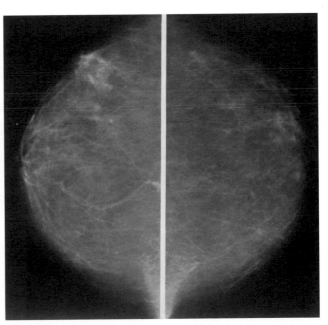

B

MA-59. Fibrosis. The focal asymmetry in the upper outer left breast on the MLO *(A)* and the CC *(B)* projections proved to be benign fibrous tissue.

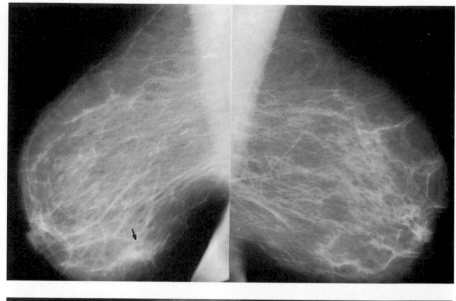

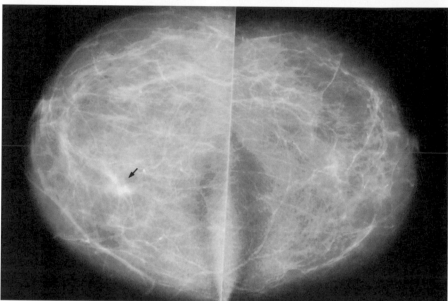

MA-60. Invasive breast cancer. The focal asymmetry *(arrow)* in the lower left breast seen on the MLO *(A)* and CC *(B)* projections was a spiculated mass on magnification and an invasive breast cancer at biopsy.

Teaching Point: Most breast cancers are first detected as focal asymmetries. It is on closer inspection that malignant characteristics are confirmed.

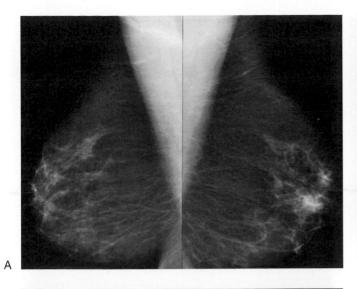

A

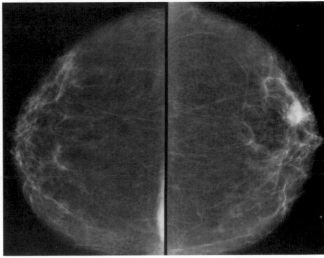

B

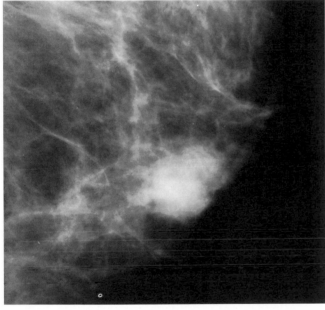

C

MA-61. Invasive breast cancer. The focal asymmetric density in the right subareolar region on the MLO *(A)* and the CC *(B)* projection is an irregular, ill-defined mass on closer inspection *(C)*. It proved to be invasive ductal carcinoma.

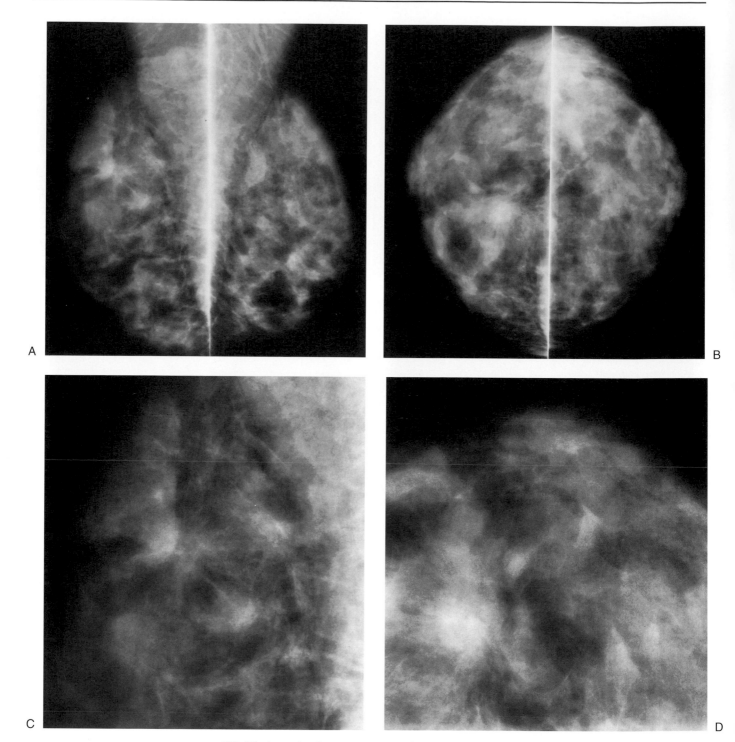

MA-62. Invasive breast cancer with an intraductal component. There is a focal asymmetry in the upper central region of the left breast seen on the MLO *(A)* and CC *(B)* projection. It becomes a spiculated mass on the magnification straight lateral *(C)* and magnification CC *(D)* projections and proved to be invasive breast cancer. An intraductal component was only evident on microscopic assessment.

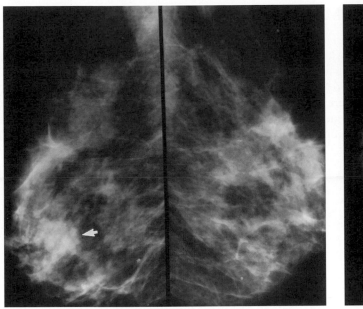
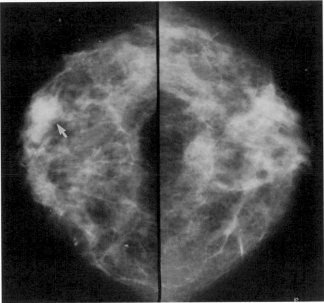

A   B

MA-63. Cancer. The focal asymmetry on the left *(arrow)* is evident on the MLO *(A)* and CC *(B)* projections. Biopsy revealed invasive ductal carcinoma.

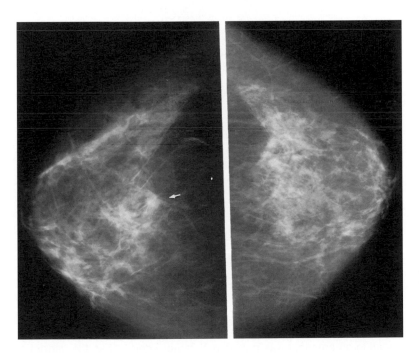

MA-64. Cancer. The focal asymmetry in the center of the left breast *(arrow)* proved to be invasive ductal carcinoma.

Teaching Point: Additional imaging is often needed to determine if a focal asymmetry represents normal tissue or a true abnormality.

ASYMMETRIC BREAST TISSUE

[See *Breast Imaging, Second Edition*, pp. 260–267.]

Asymmetric tissue density has been described as a secondary sign of malignancy, but this is true only if there is a corresponding palpable abnormality. If there is no three-dimensional density trying to form a mass, no architectural distortion, the density has not increased with time, and there are no clustered calcifications, asymmetric tissue is a normal variation. Asymmetric tissue density that has developed, however, should be viewed with some suspicion, and additional evaluation is warranted.

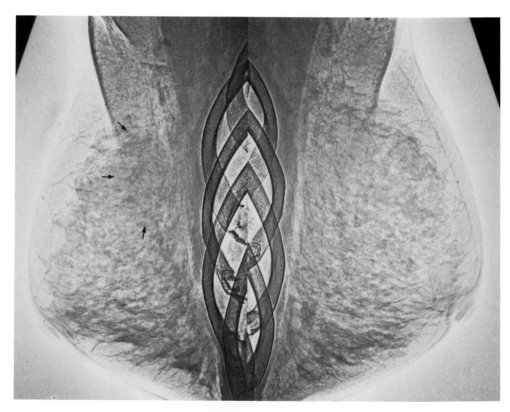

MA-65. Asymmetric tissue density that proved to be cancer. This xerogram is an example of why asymmetric tissue density was once considered a secondary sign of malignancy. The *arrows* point to an area that was palpable. It is more dense than the mirror image tissue in the opposite breast. This type of asymmetry, if not palpable, can be found with normal asymmetric breast tissue.

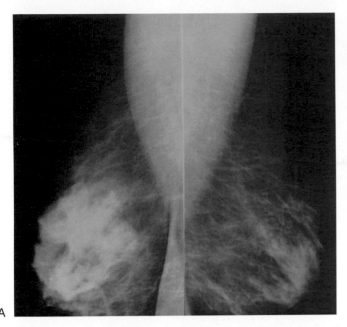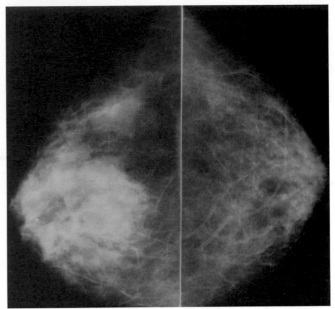

A   B

MA-66. Asymmetric breast tissue. There is pronounced asymmetric tissue involving much of the left breast on the MLO *(A)* and CC *(B)* projections. There is no architectural distortion and no mass formation. There are no calcifications and nothing is palpable. There has been no evidence of breast cancer with many years of follow-up.

Teaching Point: Asymmetric breast tissue can be pronounced, but if there is no architectural distortion and no mass formation, as well as no calcifications and nothing palpable, then it represents a normal variation.

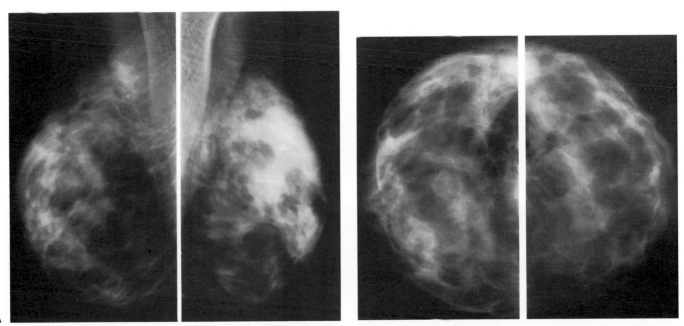

A   B

MA-67. Asymmetry due to compression differences. There is pronounced tissue density seen in the upper right breast on the MLO *(A)* projection, but not seen on the CC *(B)* views. This is an artifact of less compression on the right MLO.

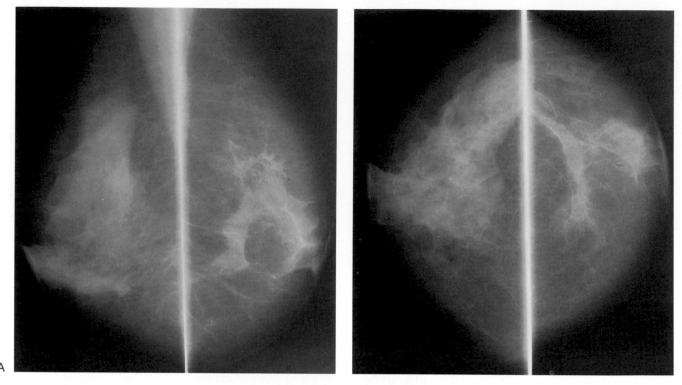

A

B

MA-68. Asymmetric tissue due to surgery on the contralateral breast. The asymmetric tissue on the left, as seen on the MLO *(A)* and CC *(B)* projections, was due to the removal of tissue from the right breast from a benign biopsy.

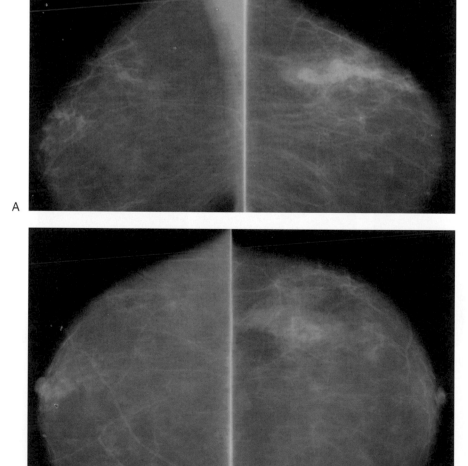

A

B

MA-69. Asymmetric breast tissue. There is asymmetric breast tissue in the upper outer right breast, as seen on the lateral *(A)* and CC *(B)* projections. Since it is not palpable, it represents a normal variation.

Teaching Point: If the normal flow of structures is not interrupted, and there is no mass or architectural distortion, this type of asymmetry is normal unless it is palpable.

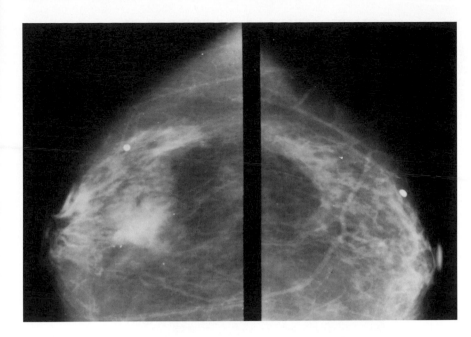

MA-70. Cancer. The asymmetry in the left breast is centrally dense. It represents a mass and not asymmetric breast tissue. It proved to be an invasive breast cancer.

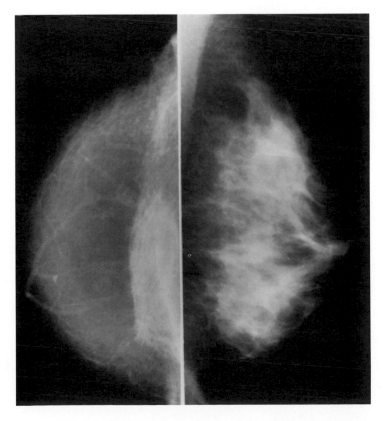

MA-71. Breast reconstruction. The right breast is normal. The left is actually a transverse rectus abdominus myocutaneous (TRAM) flap. The fat represents abdominal fat, and the muscle is part of the rectus abdominus muscle that has been moved up to the chest wall defect following a mastectomy to form a breast. The TRAM was imaged accidentally.

Teaching Point: There is no reason to routinely image a reconstructed breast.

ARCHITECTURAL DISTORTION

[See *Breast Imaging, Second Edition*, pp. 298–302.]

Architectural distortion is an important, although often subtle, sign of malignancy. The differential diagnosis includes postsurgical change and benign elastotic lesions of the breast (radial scars). When structures are pulled to a point eccentric from the nipple, cancer must be considered.

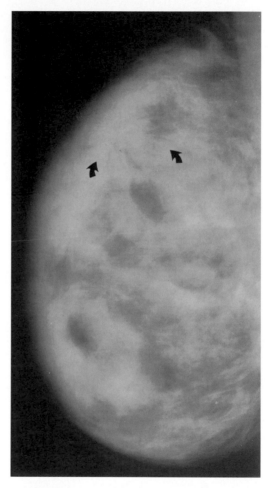

MA-72. Radial scar. The *arrows* point to an area of subtle architectural distortion in a very dense breast. It proved to be a benign elastotic lesion at biopsy.

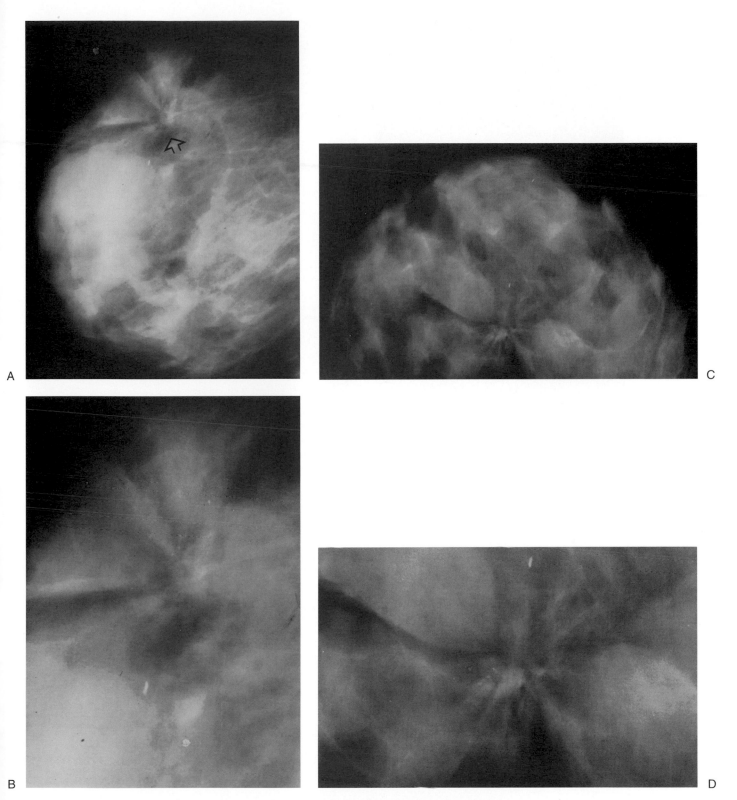

MA-73. Radial scar. The arrow points to an area of spiculated architectural distortion on the MLO *(A)* projection and enlarged *(B)* and on the CC *(C)* projection and enlarged *(D)*. There is the suggestion of a possible central mass and there are microcalcifications associated with the lesion. This very worrisome lesion proved to be a radial scar.

Teaching Point: The diagnosis can be suggested by the long spicules and absence of a mass with the suggestion of trapped fat, but biopsy is still needed to be certain that the lesion is not cancer.

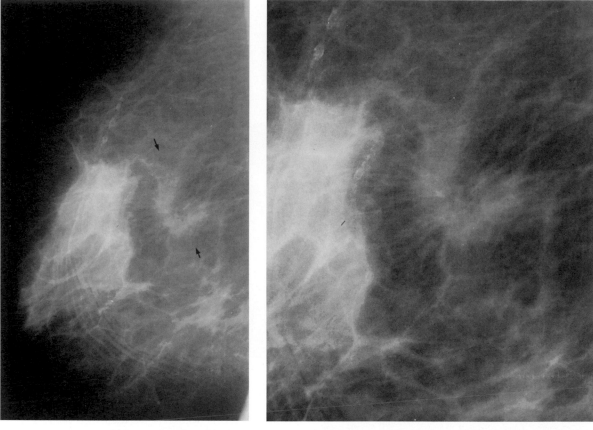

A   B

MA-74. Cancer. There is an area of architectural distortion on the MLO *(A)* and enlarged *(B)* that is partially trapping fat posteriorly and that proved to be an invasive breast cancer.

Teaching Point: Areas of architectural distortion should be biopsied, even if they seem to contain fat, unless there is a good history of a previous biopsy of a benign lesion.

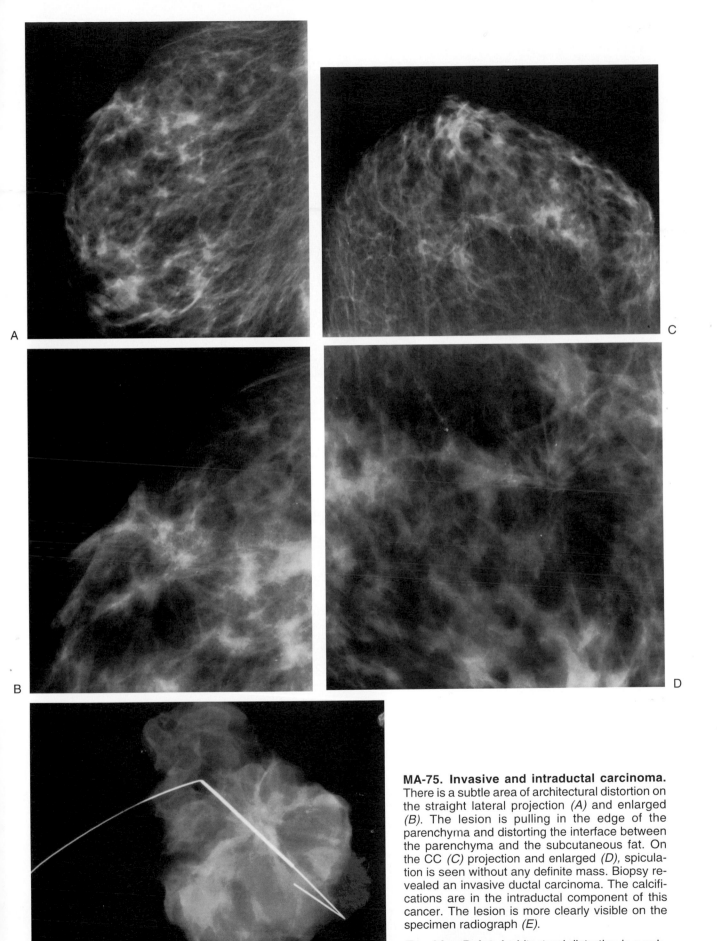

MA-75. Invasive and intraductal carcinoma.
There is a subtle area of architectural distortion on the straight lateral projection *(A)* and enlarged *(B)*. The lesion is pulling in the edge of the parenchyma and distorting the interface between the parenchyma and the subcutaneous fat. On the CC *(C)* projection and enlarged *(D)*, spiculation is seen without any definite mass. Biopsy revealed an invasive ductal carcinoma. The calcifications are in the intraductal component of this cancer. The lesion is more clearly visible on the specimen radiograph *(E)*.

Teaching Point: Architectural distortion is a subtle but important indication of possible cancer.

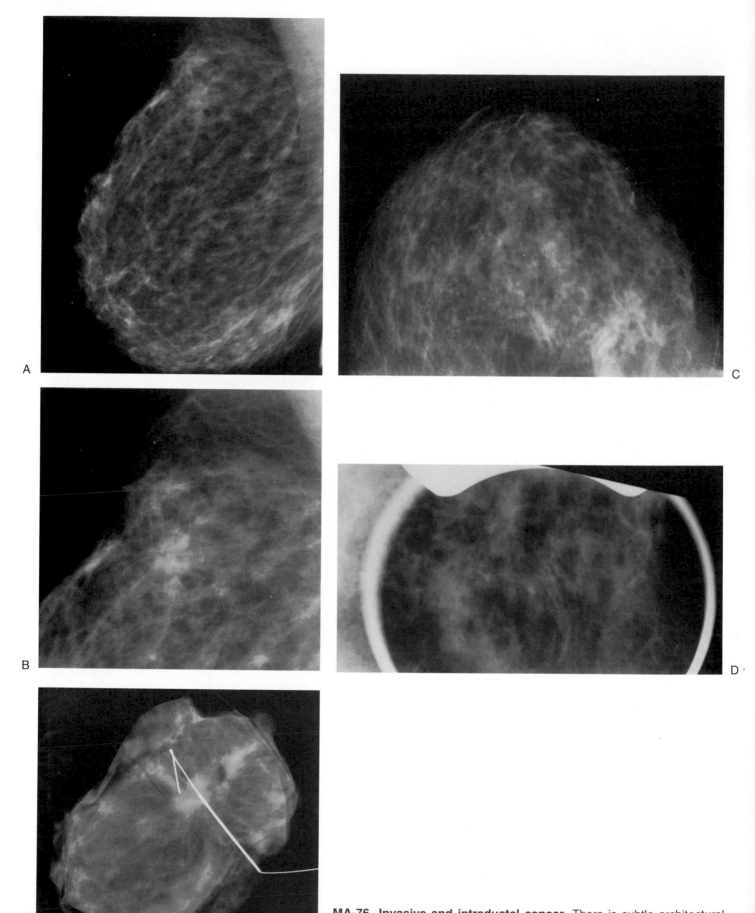

MA-76. Invasive and intraductal cancer. There is subtle architectural distortion with a possible mass seen on the MLO *(A)* and enlarged *(B)* and the CC *(C)* projection. The lesion is more apparent on the spot compression view *(D)*. Biopsy confirmed an invasive ductal carcinoma with associated DCIS *(E)*.

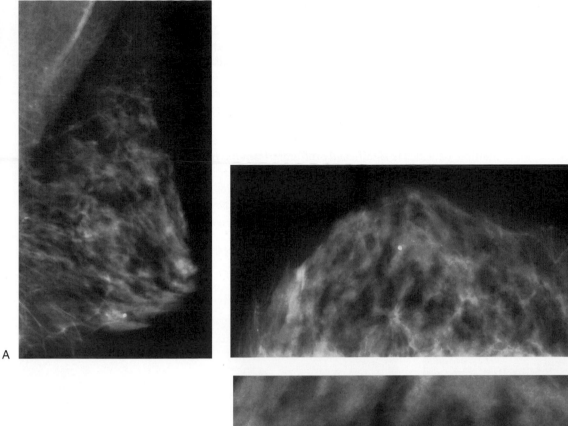

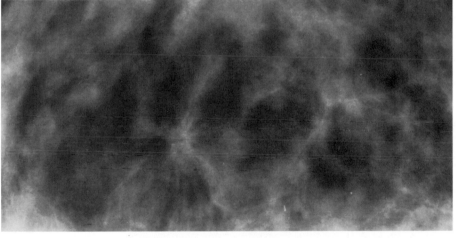

MA-77. Invasive and intraductal breast cancer. Spiculated architectural distortion is very subtle on the MLO *(A)*. It is more evident on the CC *(B)* projection, especially on the enlarged image *(C)*. Biopsy confirmed an invasive ductal carcinoma with associated intraductal tumor.

MULTIPLE DENSITIES

[See *Breast Imaging, Second Edition*, pp. 311–312.]

Multiple densities in the breasts can pose a difficult problem. When they are all similar, well circumscribed, and scattered throughout the breasts, they almost invariably represent a benign process (see the "rule of multiplicity"). The one exception to this is metastatic disease from a primary focus outside the breast to the breast, but this is extremely unusual.

Breast cancer can be multifocal, and on rare occasion multicentric, but these lesions usually have worrisome morphologic characteristics.

Breast cancer can also occur in a breast that also contains benign lesions. If one of the multiple densities is significantly different from the others, ultrasound of the questionable area is recommended (in order to determine whether it represents a cyst). Biopsy might be indicated. Multiple benign findings can obscure a more important finding.

The differential diagnosis of multiple densities seen by mammography includes skin lesions, islands of normal breast tissue, multiple cysts, multiple fibroadenomas, multiple foci of mammary carcinoma, and metastatic disease.

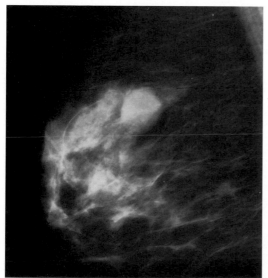

A

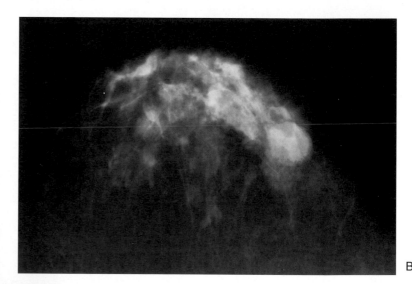

B

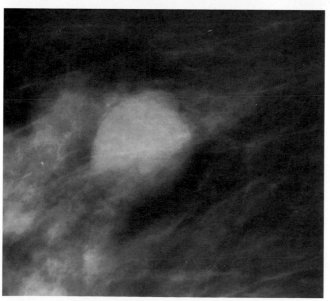

C

MA-78. Cyst. There are multiple rounded densities in the left breast as seen on the MLO *(A)* and CC *(B)* projections. The largest was of some concern due to its somewhat lobulated, obscured (or ill-defined) margin as seen on the enlarged MLO *(C)* and CC *(D)*. Ultrasound resolved the concern by revealing a simple cyst *(E)*. The other densities were smaller cysts.

Teaching Point: Ultrasound is not generally recommended for the evaluation of multiple rounded densities, but if there is an area of concern, it can be used to determine whether or not the finding represents a cyst or a solid mass.

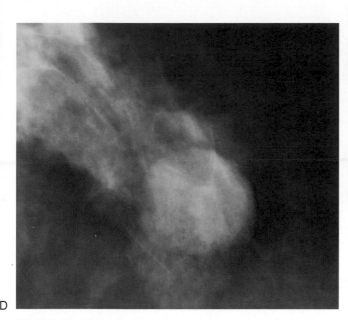

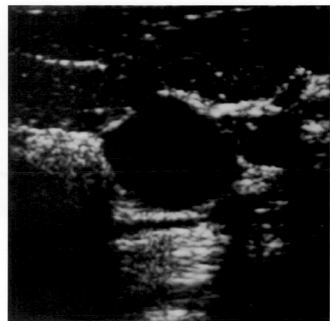

D

E

MA-78. *Continued*

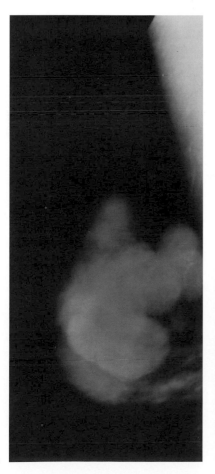

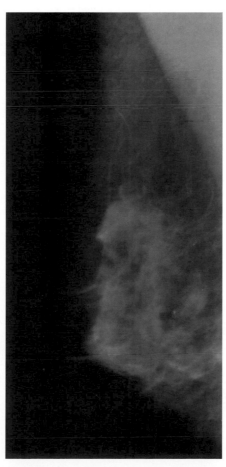

A

B

MA-79. Multiple cysts. Multiple rounded densities are evident on the lateral projection *(A)*. They were cysts by ultrasound, but the patient insisted that she wanted them all aspirated. The breast is fairly unremarkable in appearance following the aspiration of multiple cysts *(B)*.

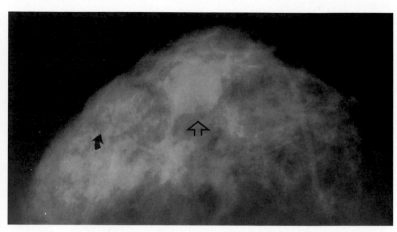

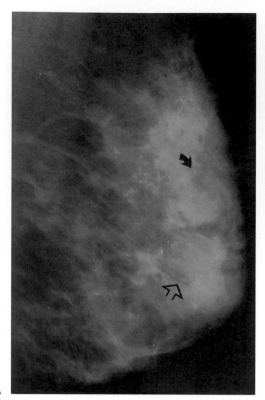

A

B

MA-80. Cyst and Fibroadenoma. There are two ovoid densities in the breast. One is in the upper *(curved arrows),* as seen on the MLO *(A),* and outer portion, as seen on the CC *(B)* projection, while the second *(open arrow)* is in the lateral subareolar region. The lateral mass proved to be a fibroadenoma, and the subareolar mass was a cyst.

Teaching Point: There is no way to differentiate these two lesions mammographically. Ultrasound could diagnose the cyst.

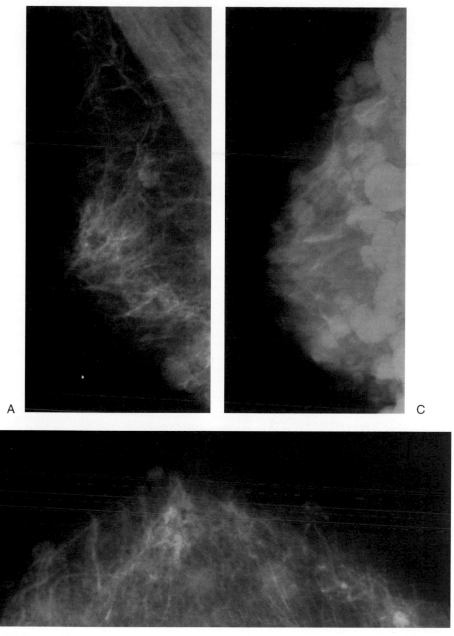

MA-81. Neurofibromatosis. Multiple densities in the skin are projected over the breast on the MLO *(A)* and CC *(B)* projections. The patient has neurofibomatosis and these are neurofibromas. This is another patient *(C)* with cutaneous neurofibromas that project over the breast.

Teaching Point: Skin lesions can project over the breast.

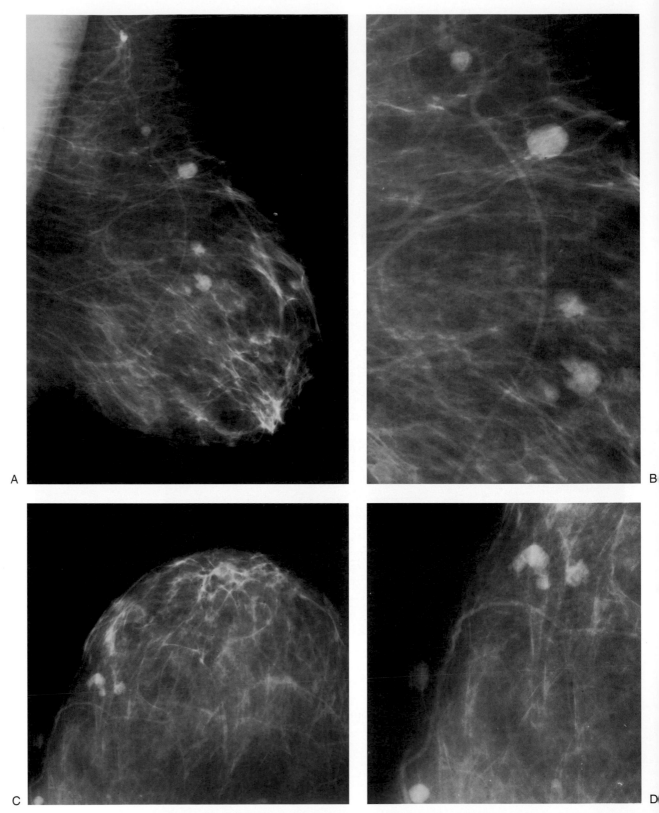

MA-82. Multiple intramammary lymph nodes. This patient had a benign, hyperplastic intramammary lymph node removed. Additional lymph nodes are visible on the MLO *(A)* and enlarged MLO *(B)* as well as on the CC *(C)* and enlarged CC *(D)*. They are in the typical location and have the typical morphology of intramammary lymph nodes.

Teaching Point: Intramammary lymph nodes are frequently multiple.

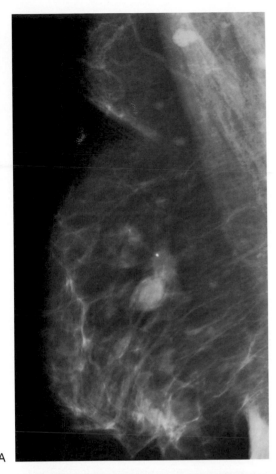

A

MA-83. Cysts and cancer. Multiple rounded densities seen on the MLO *(A)* and CC *(B)* are cysts. Immediately abutting the largest is an ill-defined mass that proved to be invasive ductal carcinoma.

Teaching Point: When there are multiple findings, look for the lesion that differs from the others.

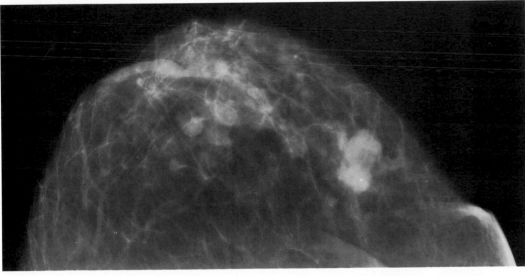

B

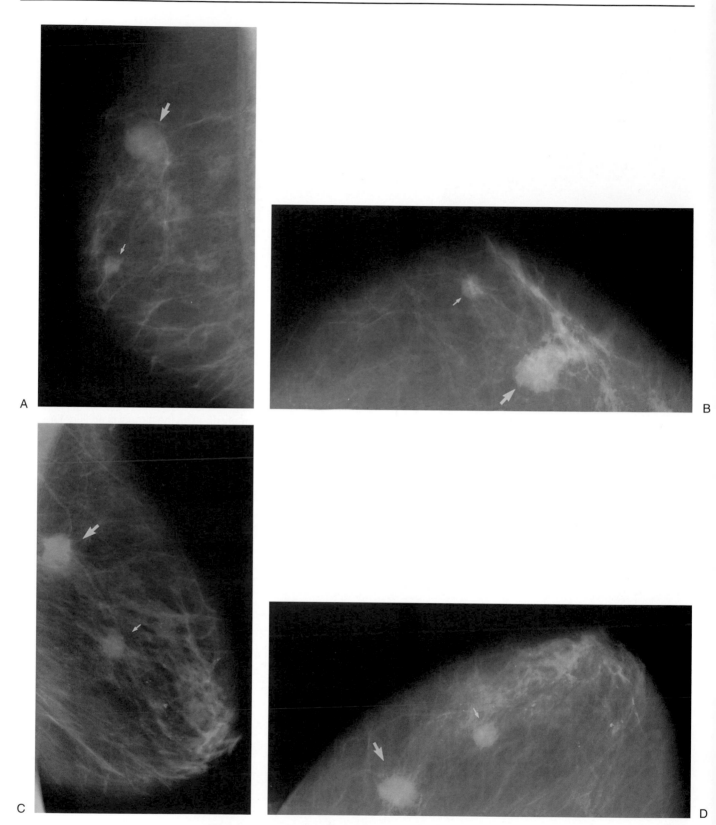

MA-84. Fibroadenomas or cancer? These lobulated, ill-defined masses on the lateral *(A)* and CC *(B)* projections of one patient that proved to be benign fibroadenomas are indistinguishable from the ill-defined masses in a second patient *(C,D)* that proved to be invasive breast cancers.

Teaching Point: Breast cancers can be multiple.

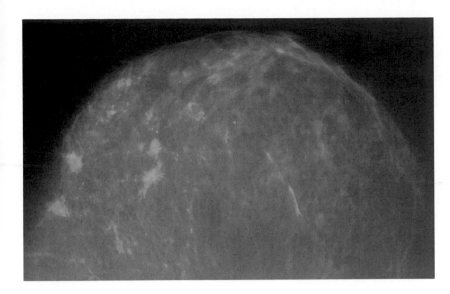

MA-85. Multifocal breast cancer. The multiple vague densities and calcifications are multifocal breast cancer.

Teaching Point: It is likely that the cancer spread intraductally throughout the segment with further genetic changes occurring independently at different points, producing invasive clones at different locations throughout the segment.

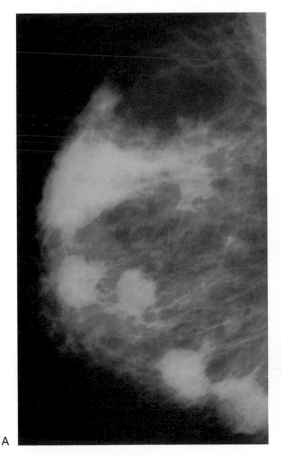
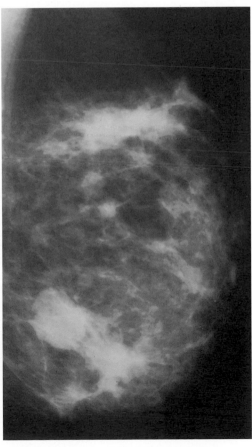

A

B

MA-86. Multifocal, bilateral breast cancer. The multiple irregular masses with ill-defined and spiculated margins on the left lateral *(A)*, right lateral *(B)*, left CC *(C)*, and right CC *(D)* are invasive breast cancers.

Teaching Point: Women with multicentric breast cancer may be genetically predisposed so that every cell in both breasts is at increased risk of malignant change.

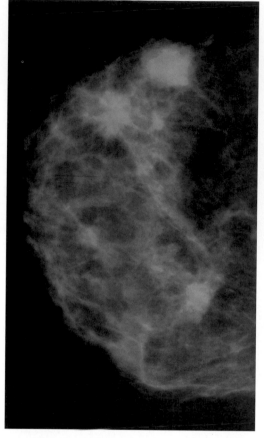

C

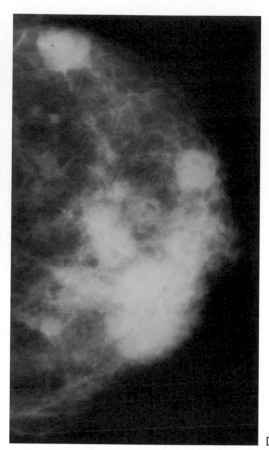

D

MA-86. *Continued*

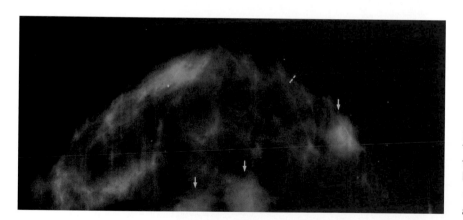

MA-87. Metastatic renal cell carcinoma. The multiple round, slightly ill-defined densities in this patient proved to be metastatic lesions from renal cell carcinoma.

Teaching Point: Metastases to the breast are often fairly well defined.

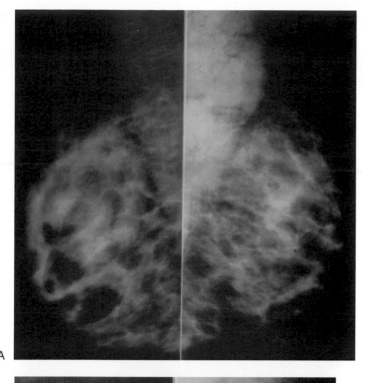

A

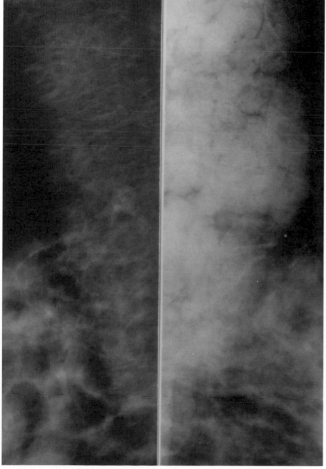

B

MA-88. Neurofibromas of the pectoralis major muscle. The rounded densities in the right breast *(A)* on close inspection *(B)* project over the pectoralis major. They are neurofibromas in this patient with neurofibromatosis.

LUCENT LESIONS AND LESIONS OF MIXED X-RAY ATTENUATION

[See *Breast Imaging, Second Edition*, pp. 355–356.]

It is extremely rare for breast cancers to contain fat. At times, a diffusely infiltrating process, such as an invasive lobular carcinoma, may infiltrate without inducing desmoplasia, and cancer cells may be interspersed with fat, but this is the exception. Encapsulated lesions that are totally radiolucent or contain islands of breast tissue are always benign. The most common form is postsurgical fat necrosis that produces "traumatic oil cysts." Lipomas and galactoceles are other causes of lucent breast lesions. The hamartoma (fibroadenolipoma) is a benign encapsulated lesion with mixed density in fat.

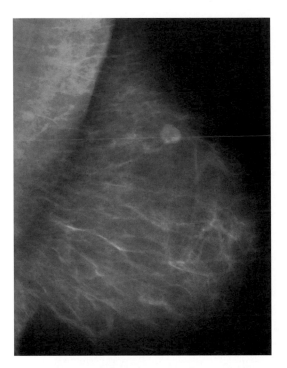

MA-89. Intramammary lymph node. The mass that has fat in its center in the upper breast, as seen on this MLO projection, is a benign intramammary lymph. [See *Breast Imaging, Second Edition,* pp. 12–13.]

Teaching Point: The most common mass in the breast that contains fat is a benign intramammary lymph node. It is usually found in the upper outer quadrant.

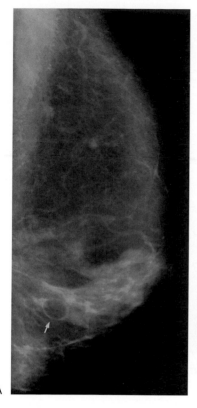

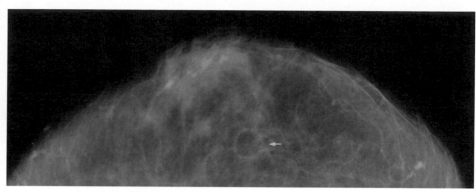

A   B

MA-90. Posttraumatic oil cyst. The encapsulated, lucent mass on the lateral *(A)* and CC *(B)* projections is a benign, postsurgical oil cyst in this patient who has had a reduction mammoplasty.

Teaching Point: Oil cysts are a form of fat necrosis in which the gelatinized fat is encapsulated and walled off as a response of the tissue to trauma.

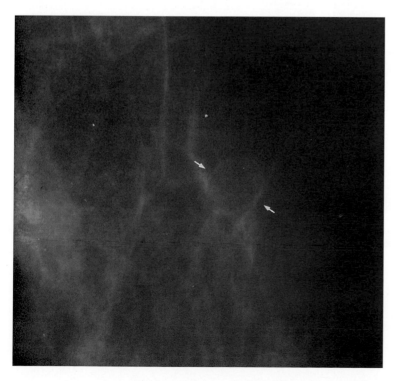

MA-91. Posttraumatic oil cyst. This oil cyst was hard on palpation, but is barely visible, and can only be seen because of its surrounding capsule.

Teaching Point: Even though they can be very firm on palpation, oil cysts may be difficult to see by mammography. Encapsulated fat, however, always indicates a benign lesion.

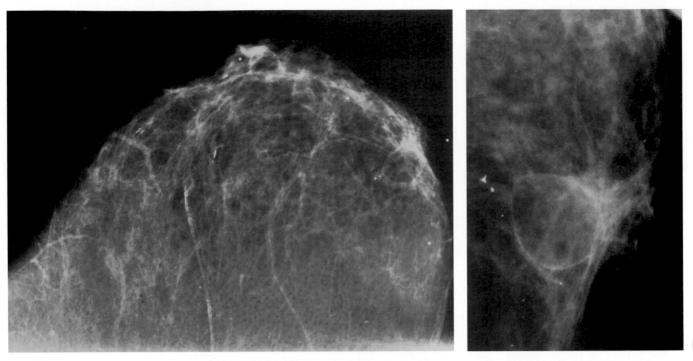

A   B

MA-92. Posttraumatic oil cyst. The palpable mass, immediately under the nipple as seen on the CC projection *(A)*, is clearly encapsulated fat on the magnification lateral image *(B)* and requires no further investigation.

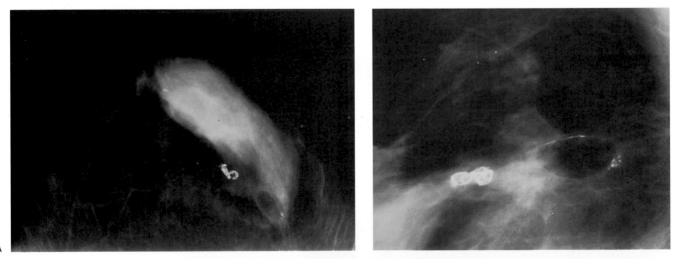

A   B

MA-93. Posttraumatic fat necrosis. In addition to the oil cyst seen posterolaterally on this CC projection *(A)*, fat necrosis has also produced the large, lucent-centered calcifications seen on the enlarged lateral projection *(B)*. The patient had undergone a reduction mammoplasty.

Teaching Point: Fat necrosis is fairly common following reduction mammoplasty.

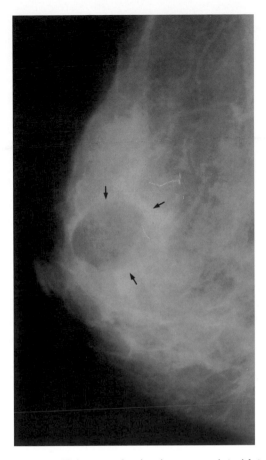

MA-94. Lipoma. This mass is clearly encapsulated fat. The patient had no history of trauma, so that it is almost certainly a benign lipoma. Regardless, no further evaluation is needed.

Teaching Point: Lipomas in the breast are likely more common than generally appreciated. Most are not visible because they are probably indistinguishable from normal intramammary fat surrounded by Cooper's ligaments.

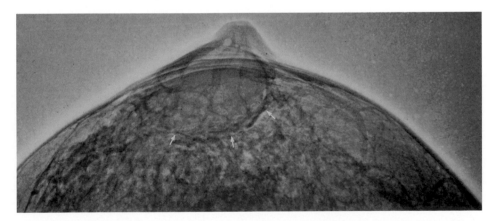

MA-95. Galactocele. The lucent lesion in the subareolar region on this positive mode xerogram is a galactocele in a woman with elevated prolactin levels.

Teaching Point: In our experience, galactoceles are extremely rare. They may be lucent if the fat content is high, of mixed density, or indistinguishable from a cyst.

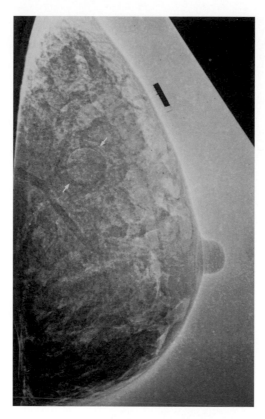

MA-96. Galactocele. This lucent lesion, seen on this positive mode lateral xerogram, was a galactocele in a lactating patient.

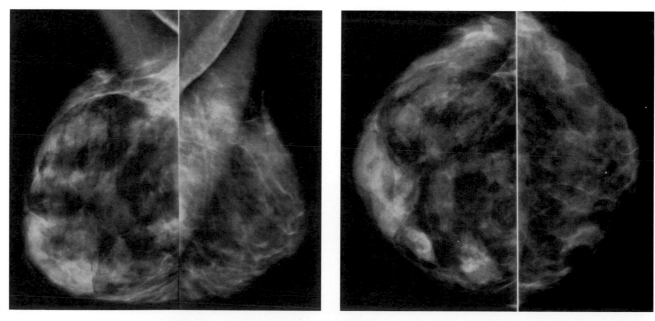

A   B

MA-97. Hamartoma. The left breast is considerably larger than the right breast due to the encapsulated mass that is of mixed density, as seen on the MLO *(A)* and CC projection *(B)*. This is the typical appearance of a mammary hamartoma, and no further investigation is indicated.

Teaching Point: If a lesion is encapsulated and contains fat, it is benign.

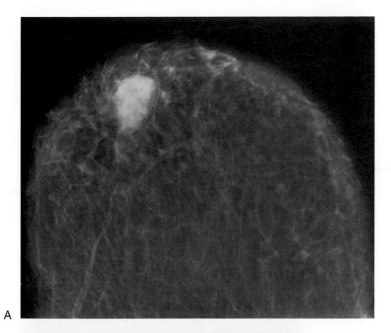

A

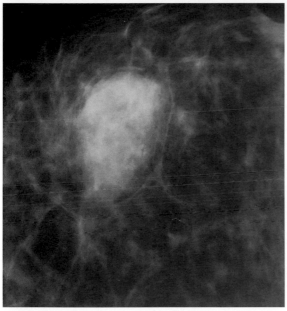

B

MA-98. Hematoma. This patient had trauma 2 weeks earlier. The mass seen on the CC *(A)* and enlarged *(B)* is of mixed density with a thin line that suggests a capsule seen because of fat on the inside. This completely resolved after several months.

Teaching Point: It is often not possible to diagnose a hematoma, but if the history is strong, and the lesion has a pseudocapsule, as seen in this case, it is reasonable to follow-up rather than intervene. The pseudocapsule may represent hemosiderin left behind as the blood is resorbed, but this is speculation.

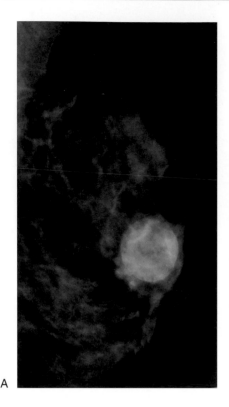

A

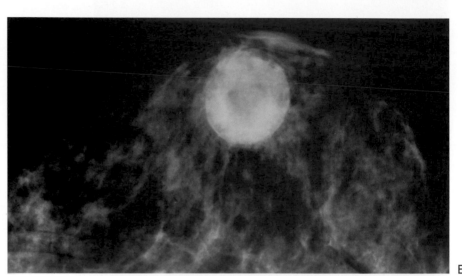

B

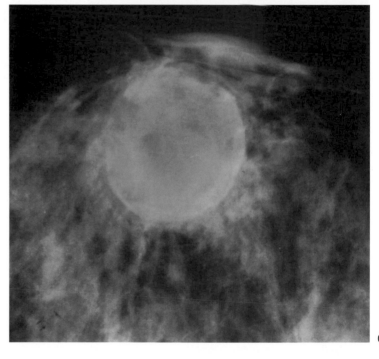

C

MA-99. Chronic hematoma. This mass appears to be calcified on the MLO *(A)*, CC *(B)*, and enlarged CC *(C)* projections, but there was no calcium at the surgical excision, requested by the patient. The density is likely due to hemosiderin left at the periphery of this incompletely resorbed hematoma from surgery several years earlier.

Teaching Point: Surgery was not needed for this lesion that was either a large mass with rim calcification, or, as demonstrated, an "encapsulated" lucent lesion. Both are benign.

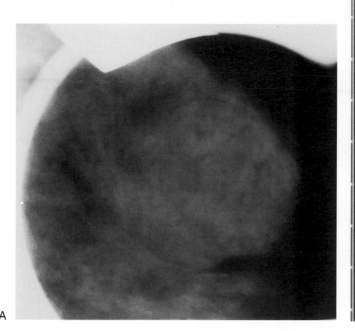

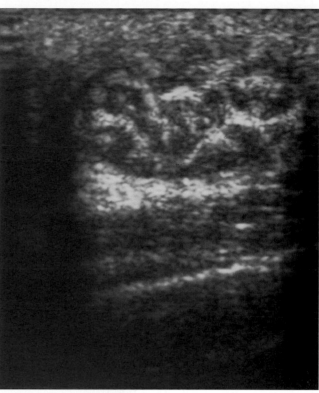

A

B

MA-100. Unusual phylloides tumor. This is a very rare phylloides tumor, seen on this spot compression CC *(A)*. Note that it contains fat in curvilinear patterns. This is reflected on the ultrasound image *(B)*, where the fat produces echogenic structures in the hypoechoic mass. This phylloides tumor contained, as part of it, elements of a well-differentiated liposarcoma.

Teaching Point: It is probably best to biopsy lesions with unusual morphology.

SKIN RETRACTION

[See *Breast Imaging, Second Edition*, pp. 342–343.]

As mammography detects smaller and earlier cancers, skin changes on mammography have become much less important. Visualization of the skin on the mammogram is not critical. Focal skin retraction is easily seen on clinical examination.

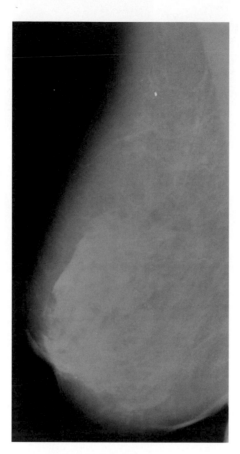

MA-101. Normal skin retraction caudal to the nipple. On this underexposed lateral, skin retraction is evident just caudal to the nipple. The same finding was present on the other side. There was no history of surgery and no cancer had developed over many years of follow-up.

Teaching Point: In some women there appears to be a normal tethering that pulls in the skin just caudal to the nipple.

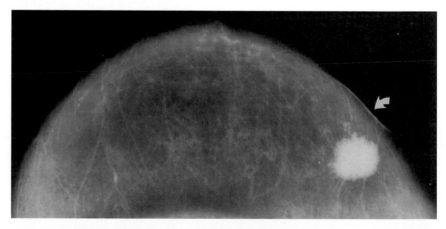

MA-102. Skin retraction due to an underlying cancer. The skin retraction that is evident on this CC projection is due to the tethering caused by the large breast cancer.

Teaching Point: Skin retraction is much less common than in the past since cancers are being found at a much smaller size and earlier stage.

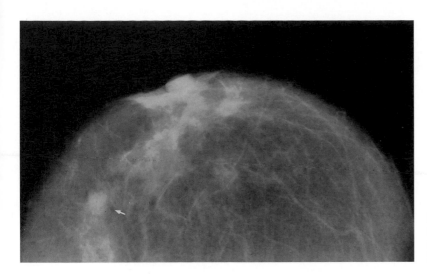

MA-103. Nipple retraction due to breast cancer. The nipple is deviated laterally, as seen on this CC projection, in the direction of the cancer in the lateral right breast.

SKIN AND TRABECULAR THICKENING

[See *Breast Imaging, Second Edition*, p. 342.]

Diffuse skin changes, associated with cancer, are late changes in the development of the tumor and are less common than in the past since more cancers are being detected at a smaller size and earlier stage. Other causes of skin and trabecular thickening include dermatologic problems such as psoriasis, inflammation, infection, and obstruction of lymphatics in the axilla or vessels in the mediastinum.

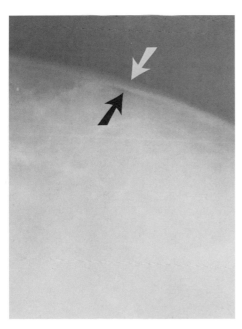

MA-104. Skin thickening due to psoriasis. The skin (between the *arrows*) was thickened due to psoriasis.

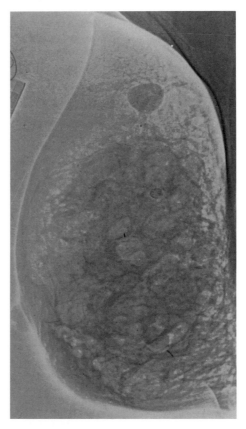

MA-105. Skin thickening due to infection. The pronounced skin thickening, particularly in the dependent portion of the left breast on this xerographic lateral image, was due to an infection. The mass high in the breast was a reactive lymph node. All resolved following a course of antibiotics.

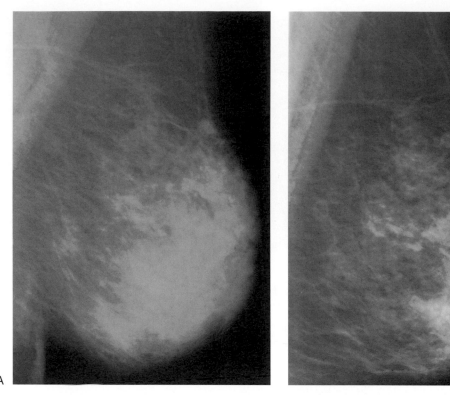

A

B

MA-106. Mastitis. This patient presented with a sore, hot, swollen breast seen on the MLO projection *(A)*. The tissues are dense (trabecular thickening) and not sharply defined, consistent with inflammation. Following antibiotic treatment, a repeat mammogram was obtained several weeks later *(B)*. The edema has resolved, providing improved mammographic detail due to better compression and elimination of the previous edema.

Teaching Point: Thickening due to mastitis is indistinguishable from that caused by a neoplastic process (see below).

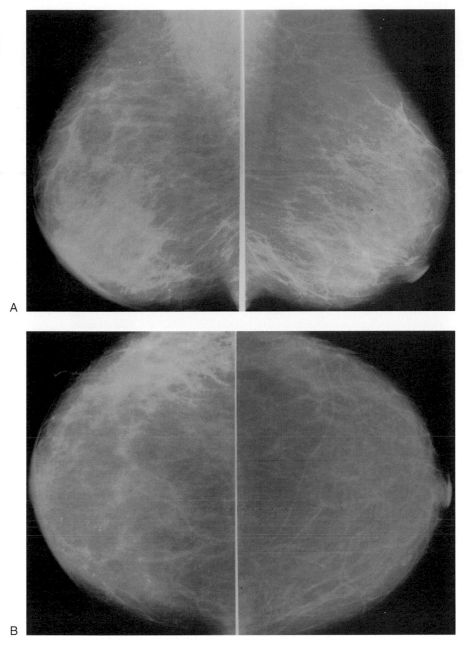

A

B

MA-107. Inflammatory cancer. The diagnosis of inflammatory cancer is made primarily on the clinical presentation (erythema, heat, and peau d'orange without a fever or elevated white blood cell count). Mammographically, as seen in the left breast of this patient with inflammatory cancer, the skin and trabecular pattern are thickened as is evident on the MLO *(A)* and CC *(B)* projections. The appearance, however, is not specific.

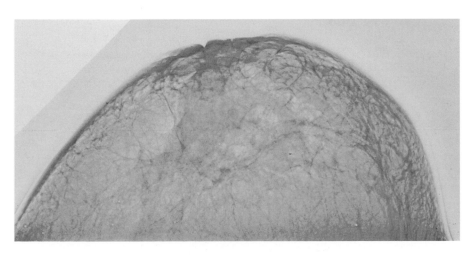

MA-108. Skin thickening due to inflammatory breast cancer. This patient presented with a 2-week history of erythema and increased heat over much of her breast. On examination the pores of the breast were accentuated by diffuse skin thickening forming what looked like the skin of an orange (peau d'orange). The positive mode xerogram clearly shows the diffuse thickening of the skin.

Teaching Point: Skin thickening is nonspecific. The diagnosis of inflammatory cancer is made based on the clinical presentation and breast biopsy.

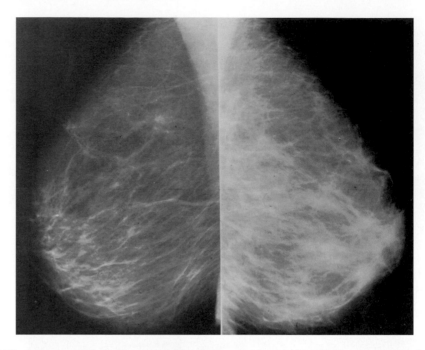

MA-109. Skin and trabecular thickening following breast irradiation. Radiation therapy for breast cancer is a common cause of skin and trabecular thickening as seen in the irradiated right breast as compared to the left.

Teaching Point: The edema following radiation therapy causes skin and trabecular thickening that may resolve over several months to several years, or become a permanent fibrotic change.

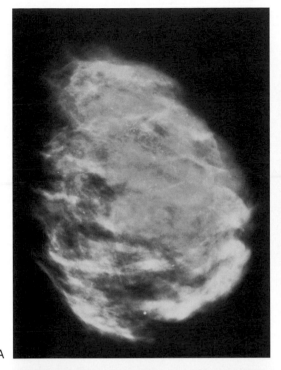

A

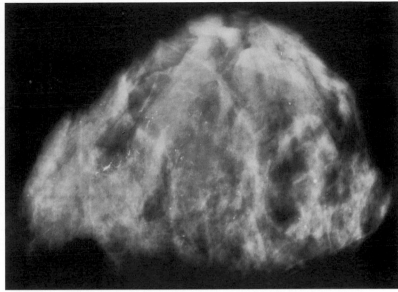

B

C

MA-110. Advanced breast cancer before and after chemotherapy. This patient presented with a breast that could not be compressed due to the large cancer occupying much of the anterior of the breast along with diffuse skin and trabecular thickening as seen on the MLO *(A)* and CC *(B)* projections. Some calcifications are barely visible. A needle biopsy confirmed the diagnosis of extensive intraductal and invasive breast cancer and the patient was placed on chemotherapy. Several months later, following a clinical response, the mammogram was repeated *(C)*. The edema has diminished, although there is still some skin thickening, and the calcifications of necrotic intraductal cancer are clearly evident.

Teaching Point: Advanced breast cancers may demonstrate a response on the mammogram to primary chemotherapy. Calcifications may increase, decrease, or remain the same. Unfortunately, they cannot be used to determine the viability of residual cancer.

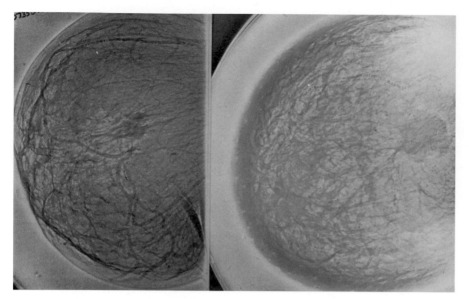

MA-111. "Neglected" breast cancer. This patient had refused treatment for the cancer detected in the left breast *(left image)*. She returned 3 years later with a much larger tumor, and diffuse skin and trabecular thickening, as seen on this positive mode xerogram due to lymphatic involvement.

Teaching Point: Neglected breast cancer differs from inflammatory breast cancer. Inflammatory cancer is generally more aggressive and progresses more rapidly.

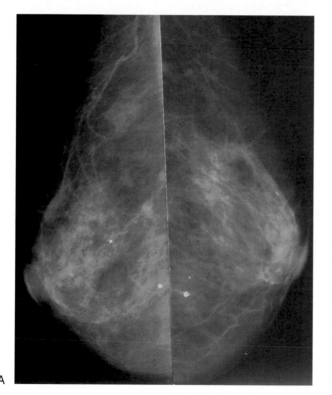

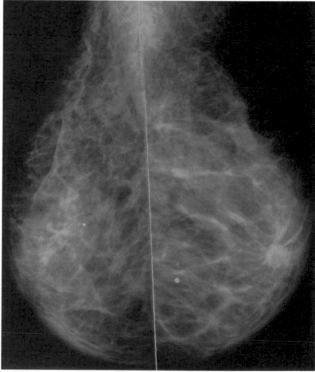

A   B

MA-112. Superior vena caval obstruction. This patient had superior vena caval obstruction from what proved to be lung cancer causing her to go from normal-appearing mammograms *(A)* to diffuse skin and trabecular thickening *(B)* over the course of several months.

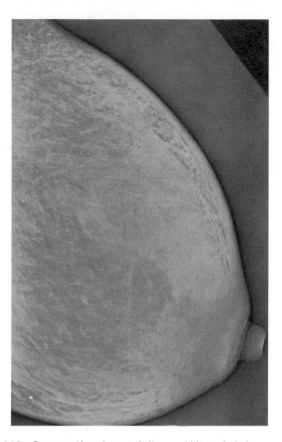

MA-113. Congestive heart failure. Although it is uncommon, edema of the breast can be caused by cardiac "obstruction," as in this patient whose negative mode xerogram shows pronounced skin and trabecular thickening that was due to her congestive heart failure.

Teaching Point: Skin and trabecular thickening can be due to lymphatic engorgement in the breast, obstruction of the lymphatics in the axilla, or more central obstruction to lymphatic or venous flow.

THE AXILLA

[See *Breast Imaging, Second Edition*, p. 231.]
Mammography is not very useful in evaluating the axilla, but benign and malignant conditions may be seen on the axillary portion of the image.

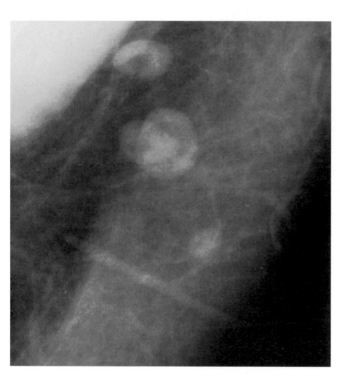

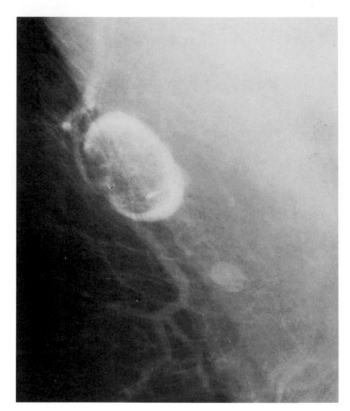

MA-114. Normal axillary lymph nodes. Axillary nodes typically are round, oval, or reniform as seen on this enlarged axillary portion of this MLO projection of the right breast.

Teaching Point: Axillary lymph nodes that do not contain fat may be as large as 1.5 to 2.0 cm. If they are larger, and do not contain fat, pathology should be suspected.

MA-115. Normal axillary lymph node. Axillary lymph nodes frequently contain a large amount of fat as seen on this enlargement of the axillary portion of the MLO projection of the left breast.

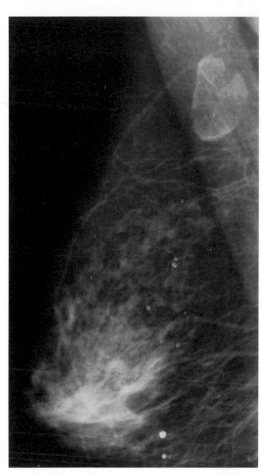

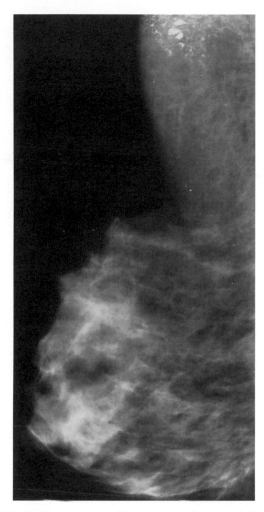

MA-116. Normal axillary lymph node. Although it is very large, this axillary lymph node is not abnormal since its size is due to the large amount of fat contained within it.

Teaching Point: Axillary lymph nodes may become very large. As long as their size is due to large amounts of fat, they are considered normal.

MA-117. Antiperspirant. What appear to be calcifications projected over the axilla of the left breast, on this MLO projection, are actually antiperspirant on the skin.

Teaching Point: Antiperspirant, but not deodorant, will show up as pseudocalcifications.

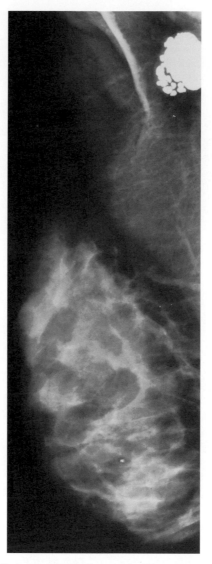

MA-118. Calcified lymph node. The densely calcified lymph node in the left axilla of this 34-year-old woman, seen on this MLO projection, was palpable.

Teaching Point: Densely calcified axillary lymph nodes have no known significance. If the calcifications are small, fine deposits, then metastatic breast cancer should be suspected, but this is extremely rare.

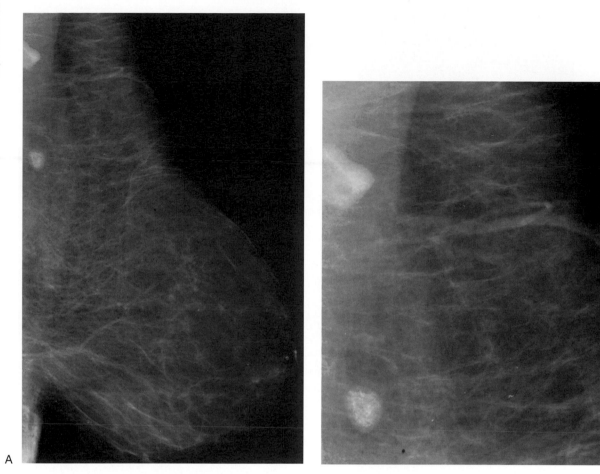

A   B

MA-119. Intranodal gold deposits. What appear to be punctate calcifications seen in the lymph nodes of the axilla on the MLO *(A)* and enlarged *(B)* are actually particles of gold secondary to injections that the patient had received for her rheumatoid arthritis.

Teaching Point: The fact that the deposits are extremely small, yet highly attenuating, should raise the correct suspicion that they represent a heavy metal.

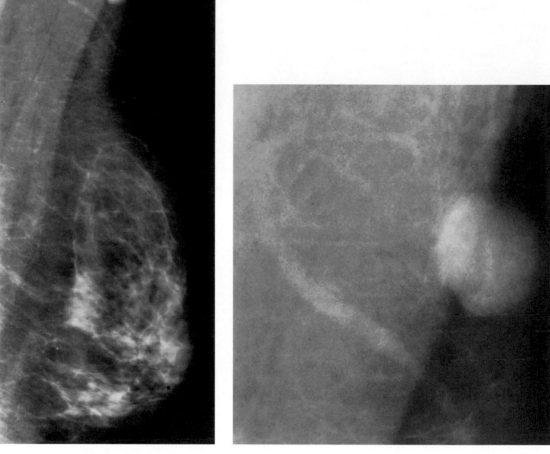

MA-120. Apocrine hydrocystoma. The mass that is visible in the axilla on the MLO *(A)* is seen enlarged *(B)*. It cannot be considered a normal lymph node since it is not reniform and does not contain fat, and has a microlobulated margin that raises some concern. Some calcifications may also be present. Biopsy revealed a benign skin cyst.

Teaching Point: Not all axillary masses are lymph nodes.

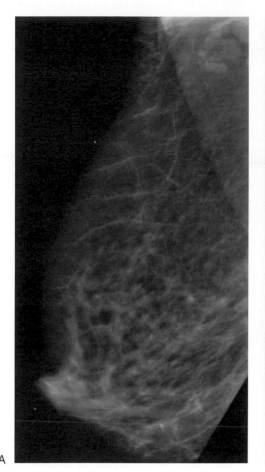
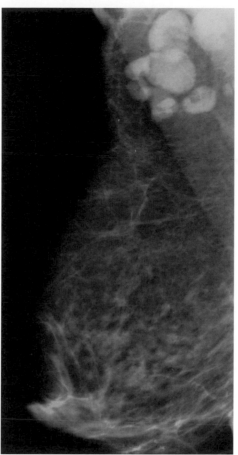

A   B

MA-121. Lymphoma. The axillary lymph nodes as seen on this first MLO *(A)* are normal. They became enlarged without containing fat *(B)*, and biopsy revealed lymphoma.

Teaching Point: Solid lymph nodes that are larger than 1.5 to 2.0 cm should be considered abnormal.

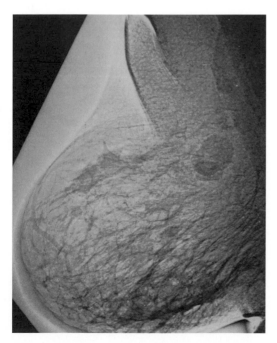

MA-122. Breast cancer with metastasis to an axillary tail lymph node. There is a cancer in the lower portion of the left breast as seen on this positive mode xerogram in the lateral projection. The mass is due to metastatic disease to a lymph node in the axillary tail of the breast. Skin thickening is due to obstruction of the axillary lymphatics from tumor.

Teaching Point: Metastatic disease to the axilla may be visible on a mammogram, but the absence of visibly abnormal lymph nodes does not exclude nodal involvement.

Section IV:
Unusual Lesions

There are findings and lesions that can be seen on mammography that are extremely rare. The figures in this section are a sampling of some of the unusual lesions that we have seen.

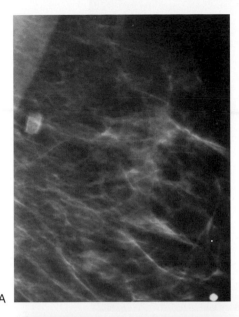

A

UN-1. Hickman catheter sleeve. The cylindrical structure on the MLO *(A)* and CC *(B)* projections is the sleeve through which a catheter had been passed as part of a chemotherapy delivery system. Since the sleeve is sutured beneath the skin, it is frequently left behind when the catheter is removed.

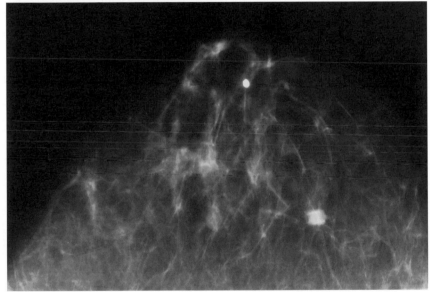

B

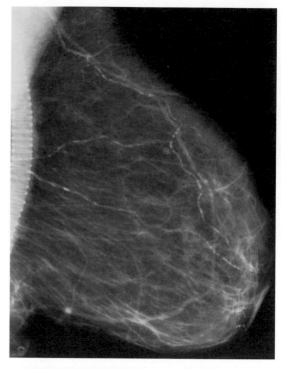

UN-2. Axillofemoral graft. The tubular structure at the back of the breast was actually lateral to it. It is the support structure of an axillofemoral graft that had been placed to correct problems from vascular occlusive disease.

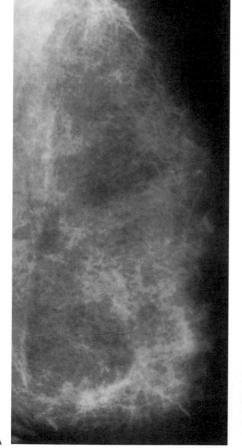

A

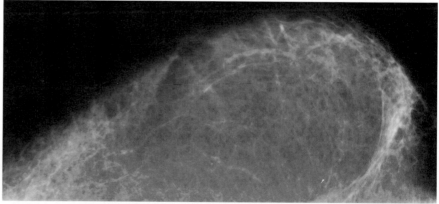

B

UN-3. Transverse rectus abdominus myocutaneous (TRAM) flap. The patient insisted on a mammogram of her reconstructed right breast. This is nothing more than the fat of the lower abdomen that has been moved through a subcutaneous tunnel to fill the space from which the right breast had been removed. At the back is the muscular (atrophying) backing through which the graft receives its blood supply as seen on the lateral *(A)* and CC *(B)* projections. There is generally no reason to perform a mammogram if there is no native breast tissue remaining.

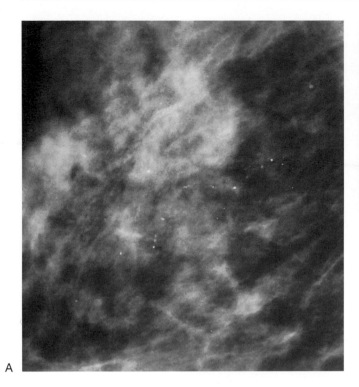

A

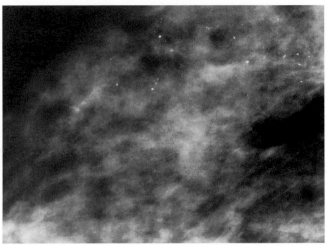

B

UN-4. Bullet fragments. These extremely high attenuation particles (dense for their very small size) seen on the enlarged MLO *(A)* and CC *(B)* projections are clearly metallic and were due to a bullet that passed through the lateral left breast many years earlier.

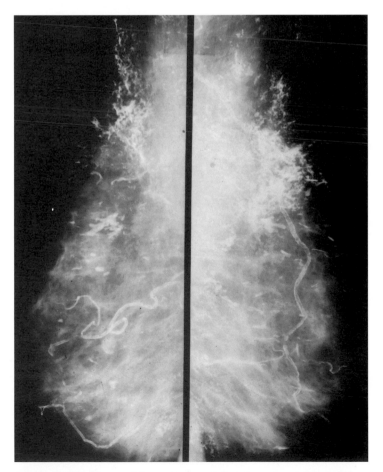

UN-5. Scleroderma. These large calcifications are subcutaneous and in a patient with scleroderma. There is virtually no other diagnosis for this pattern of calcium deposition.

Section V:
Ultrasound Atlas

Breast ultrasound is primarily useful for cyst/solid differentiation, and for guiding needle procedures. Although, on a statistical basis, most solid masses in the breast are benign, ultrasound is less accurate than tissue diagnosis in differentiating benign from malignant lesions. Some 25% to 35% of breast cancers produce posterior acoustic shadowing. Most breast cancers have a length to height ratio that is less than 1.4, and many are oriented with their long axis perpendicular to the skin. However, breast cancer can be elongated parallel to the skin, can appear sharply marginated with a homogeneous internal echo texture, and can demonstrate retrotumoral acoustic enhancement.

Internal echoes are extremely important in differentiating cystic from solid lesions, and careful evaluation of a given lesion and proper gain settings are necessary to avoid suppressing important internal echoes. [See *Breast Imaging, Second Edition,* pp. 409–443.]

CYSTS

[See *Breast Imaging, Second Edition,* p.427]

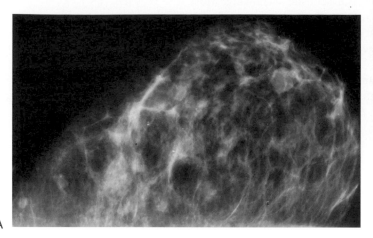

A

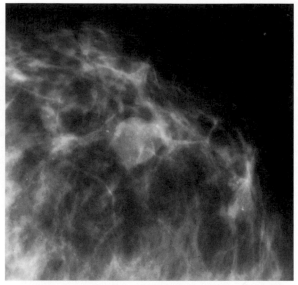

B

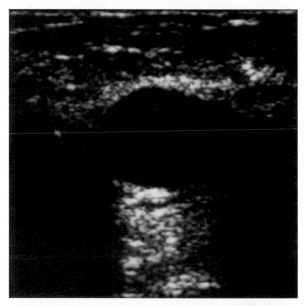

C

US-1. Cyst. The mass in the anterior medial right breast on the CC projection *(A)* is low in x-ray attenuation and round with an obscured margin on the enlarged view *(B).* Ultrasound demonstrated an anechoic mass that is round, with enhanced through transmission of sound *(C).* The patient wished confirmation so the cyst was aspirated. A small amount of air was introduced demonstrating the cyst on the CC projection *(D)* and enlarged *(E).*

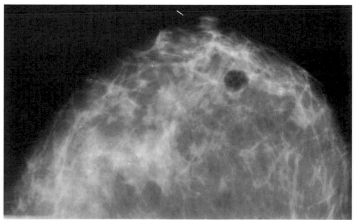

D

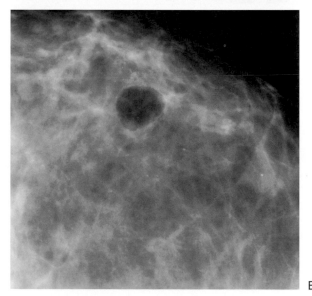

E

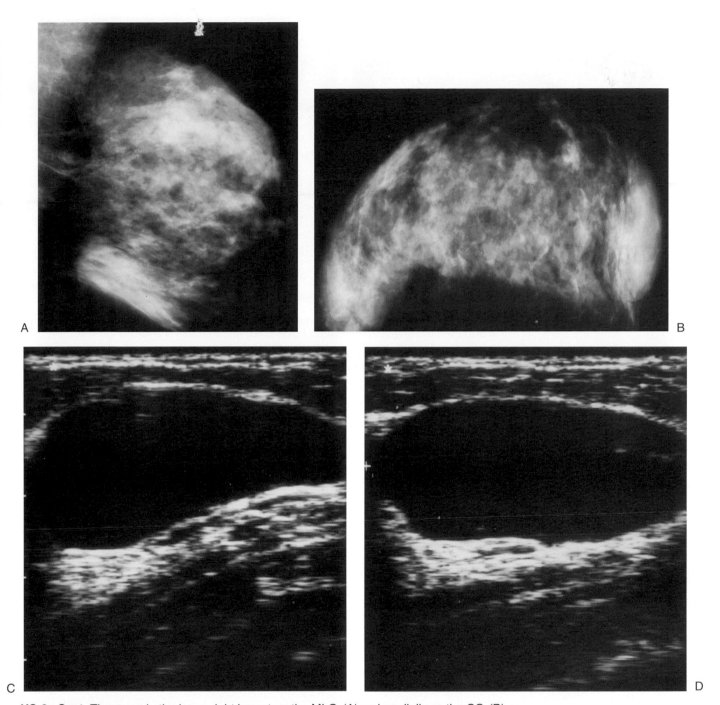

US-2. Cyst. The mass in the lower right breast on the MLO *(A)* and medially on the CC *(B)* projections in this 40-year-old woman proved, on ultrasound, to be a large, nondistended cyst on sagittal *(C)* and transverse *(D)* scans.

Teaching Point: Cysts may be tense and distended or soft and patulous.

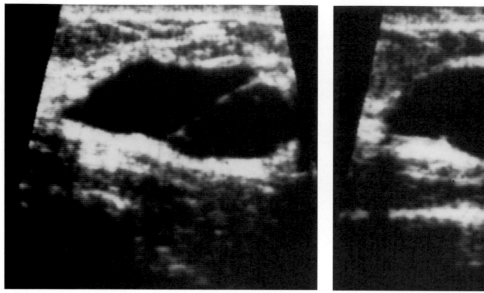

A   B

US-3. Cyst. This cyst appears to be septated in one scan plane *(A)*, but in the other plane it is apparent that the cyst is merely lobulated *(B)* and that this is a fold in the wall.

Teaching Point: Cysts are usually dilated lobules, and they may retain some of the shape of the lobule.

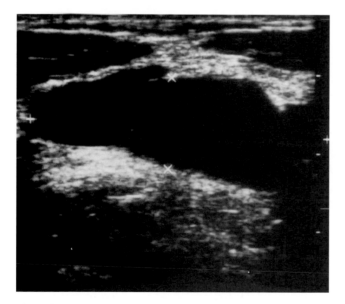

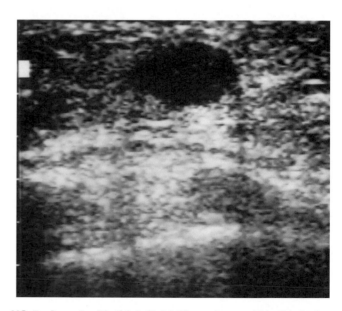

US-4. Septated cyst. This is another example of a benign "septated cyst."

Teaching Point: Septations are almost always due to the retention of the acinar structure as the lobule dilates. Septations are not a reason for concern.

US-5. A cyst with thick fluid. The echoes within this lesion made it indeterminate by ultrasound. Under ultrasound guidance, thick, mucous-like yellow fluid was removed and the cyst resolved.

Teaching Point: A cyst with internal echoes can be difficult to differentiate from a solid mass. When in doubt, aspiration can easily resolve the question.

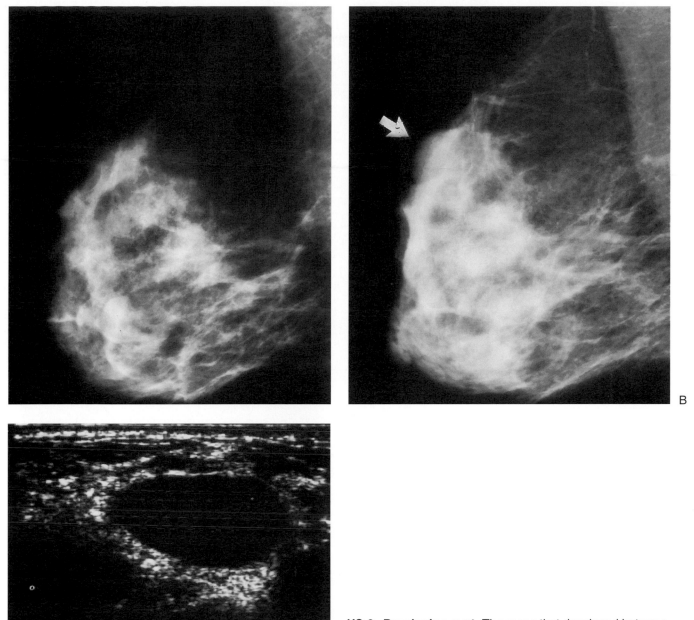

US-6. Developing cyst. The mass that developed between the first MLO *(A)* and the second *(B)* appeared as a bulge in the anterior, superior left breast. It was easily diagnosed as a cyst by ultrasound *(C)*.

INTRACYSTIC LESIONS

[See *Breast Imaging, Second Edition,* pp. 285–286, 428–429, 517–518.]

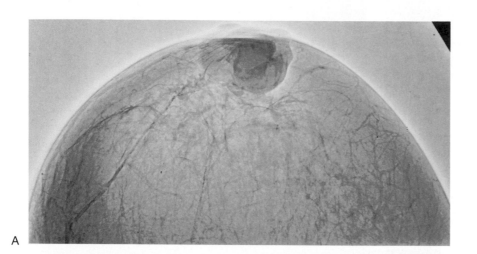

A

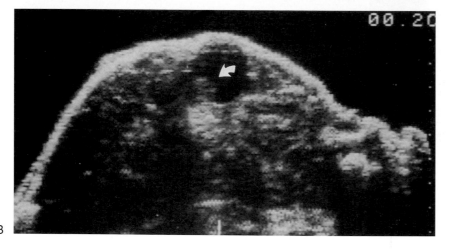

B

US-7. Intracystic papilloma. The subareolar duct is cystically dilated as seen on this CC xerogram *(A)*. The whole breast ultrasound slice demonstrates the intracystic mass *(B)* that proved to be a benign papilloma.

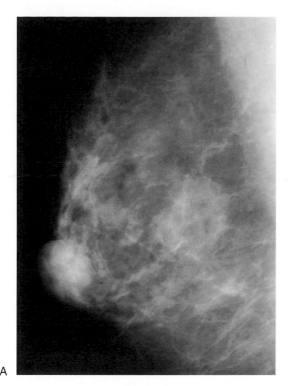

A

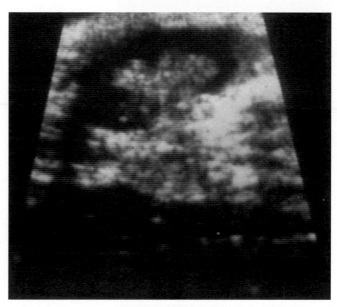

B

US-8. Intraductal papilloma. Although the lateral mammogram only demonstrates a lobulated subareolar mass *(A)*, the ultrasound *(B)* shows the intracystic mass and the fronds of
what proved to be a benign intraductal papilloma.

Teaching Point: Although ultrasound can reveal intracystic masses, benign cannot be differentiated from malignant without a biopsy.

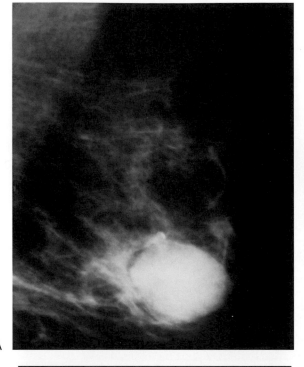

A

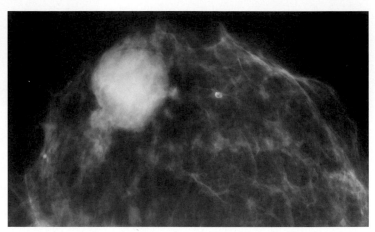

B

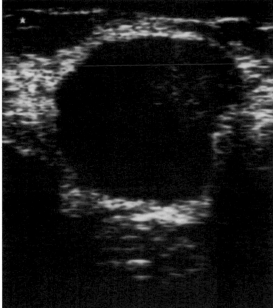

C

US-9. Intracystic papilloma. The lobulated mass on the MLO *(A)* and CC *(B)* projections was found to contain a mass in the wall by ultrasound *(C)* that proved to be an intracystic papilloma.

Teaching Point: Benign intracystic lesions cannot be differentiated from malignant ones. A tissue diagnosis is needed.

HYPOECHOIC MASSES

[See *Breast Imaging, Second Edition,* pp. 431, 437.]

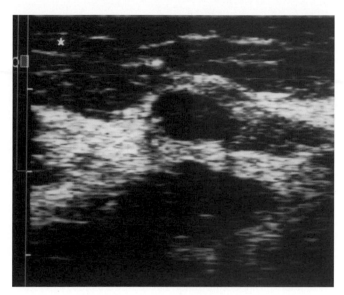

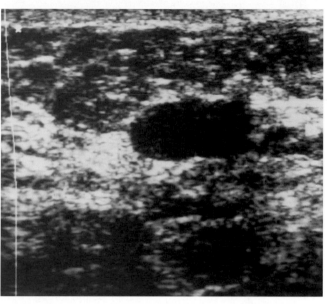

US-10. Fibroadenoma. This hypoechoic mass is oval in shape with low-level internal echoes. The tissue behind the mass is isoechoic.

Teaching Point: The histology cannot be determined. Ultrasound only determines that it is a solid mass.

US-11. Fibroadenoma. The mass is lobulated and hypoechoic with some slight reduction in the through transmission of sound.

Teaching Point: Most fibroadenomas are elongated. Unfortunately, some cancers are also elongated.

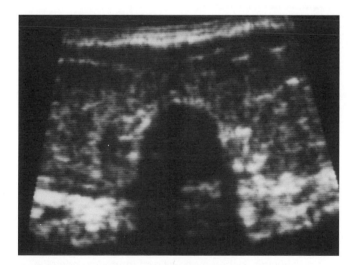

US-12. Fibroadenoma. This fibroadenoma has only low-level internal echoes. It is round with posterior acoustic shadowing.

Teaching Point: Although most fibroadenomas are elongated, some, such as this lesion, are not. This lesion is indistinguishable from breast cancer.

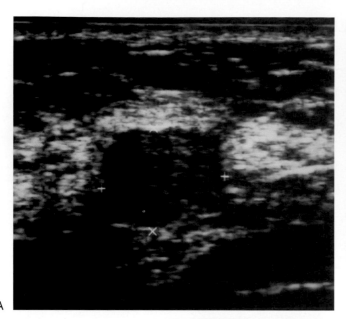
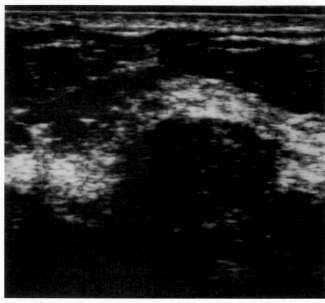

A   B

US-13. Fibroadenoma. This palpable mass was not visible by mammography due to the dense surrounding breast tissue. The mass is ovoid in shape, as seen on the transverse *(A)* and longitudinal *(B)* images. Its margins are fairly smooth with some lobulations. It is hypoechoic with a uniform echo texture. Parts of the tumor transmit sound, while other parts reduce the through transmission of sound. Ultrasound-guided core needle biopsy revealed a fibroadenoma.

Teaching Point: In young women (under the age of 35), any solid mass is almost certainly a fibroadenoma on a statistical basis. However, given that benign and malignant solid masses cannot be reliably differentiated by ultrasound, and the ease and safety of a breast biopsy, we favor a tissue diagnosis.

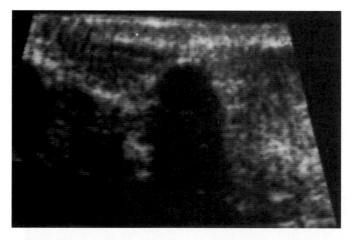

US-14. Oil cyst. This round mass is almost anechoic and causes posterior acoustic shadowing. By mammography it was a radiolucent posttraumatic oil cyst formed by necrosis.

Teaching Point: Oil cysts are so characteristic on mammography that there is no reason to use ultrasound in their evaluation. This was obtained only out of scientific interest.

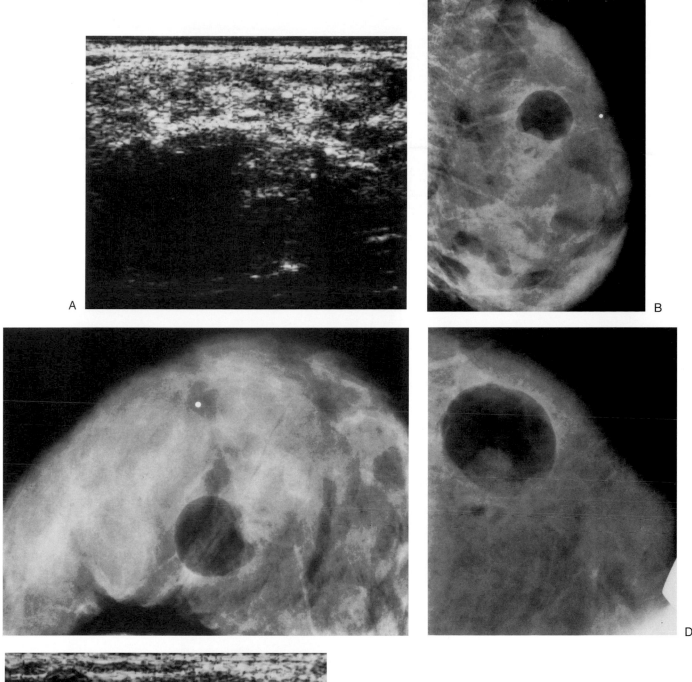

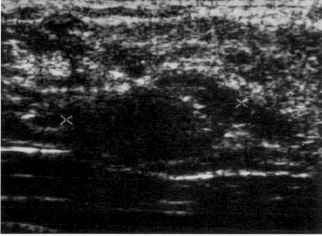

US-15. Galactocele and a fibroadenoma (contributed by Norman Sadowsky, M.D.). A lobulated mass appears to have cystic and solid components on ultrasound *(A)*. It was aspirated, and milky material was withdrawn. Air was introduced, and the MLO *(B)* and CC *(C)* projections were obtained. They show a cyst containing the air. There appears to be a mass in the cyst *(D)* that is solid on the follow-up ultrasound *(E)*. This proved to be a fibroadenoma.

Teaching Point: More than one process can occur.

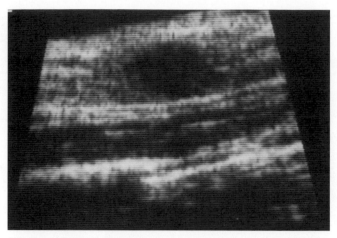

US-16. Invasive breast cancer. This mass is oval, but has ill-defined margins and contains low-level internal echoes. It proved to be a 1-cm invasive ductal carcinoma.

Teaching Point: Solid masses that are ill-defined by ultrasound are suspicious.

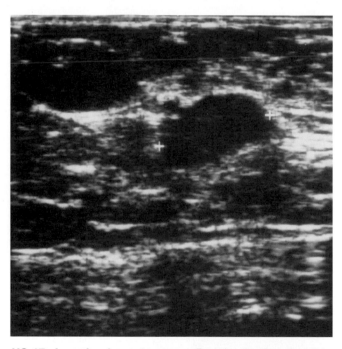

US-17. Invasive breast cancer. Despite the fact that this slightly lobulated, hypoechoic mass is elongated and the retrotumoral tissues are isoechoic, it proved to be an invasive breast cancer and, unfortunately, an axillary lymph node was positive.

Teaching Point: Although there are some morphologic criteria that work most of the time to differentiate benign from malignant masses, for a given lesion ultrasound cannot accurately make the differentiation, and biopsy is indicated.

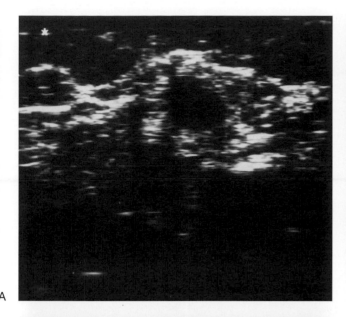

A

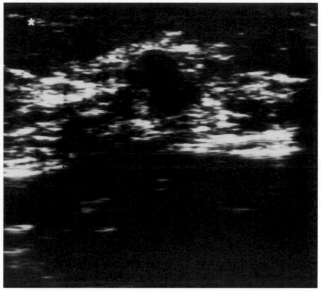

B

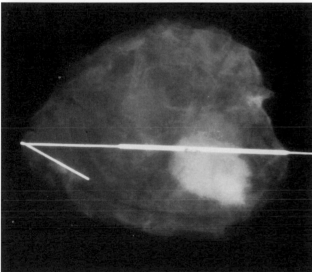

C

US-18. Invasive ductal carcinoma. This mass could be mistaken for a small cyst *(A)*, but additional imaging reveals a "dumbbell"-shaped mass *(B)* that is clearly more irregular on the specimen radiograph *(C)* than the ultrasound indicated.

Teaching Point: The entire lesion must be evaluated. Ultrasound must be used with caution.

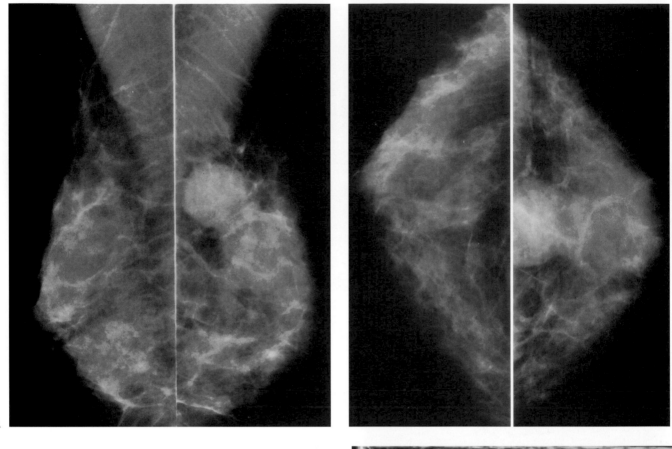

A

B

US-19. Grade III invasive ductal carcinoma. This palpable mass in the right breast of a 36-year-old woman is fairly well-defined on the MLO *(A)* and CC *(B)* projections with obscured margins. On the transverse scan *(C)* it is lobulated with a heterogeneous internal echo texture with possible cystic or necrotic spaces. Although its mammographic appearance and the patient's age suggest a possible fibroadenoma, it proved to be an invasive breast cancer with multiple positive axillary lymph nodes.

Teaching Point: A heterogeneous internal echotexture should raise the level of concern.

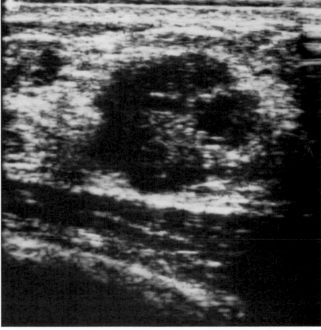

C

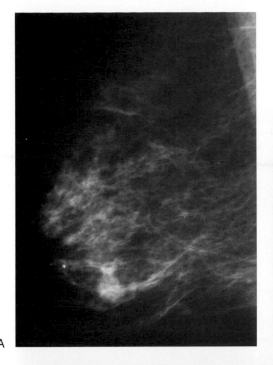

A

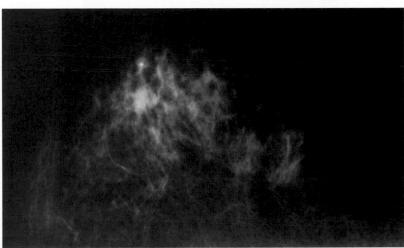

B

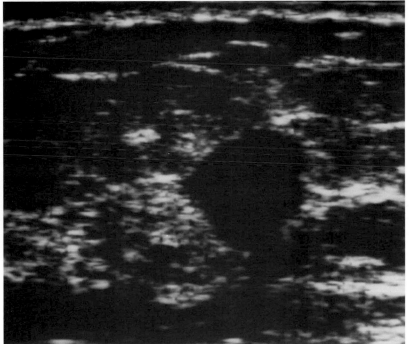

C

US-20. Invasive ductal carcinoma. The clinically occult, ill-defined mass on the MLO *(A)* and CC *(B)* projections is irregular in shape on ultrasound *(C)*, is "vertically oriented," and contains low-level internal echoes. Ultrasound-guided core needle biopsy revealed invasive ductal carcinoma.

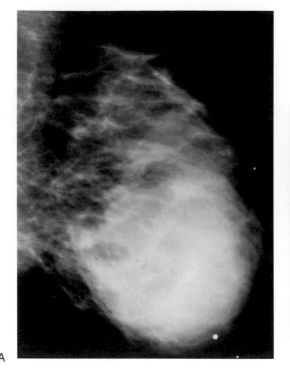

A

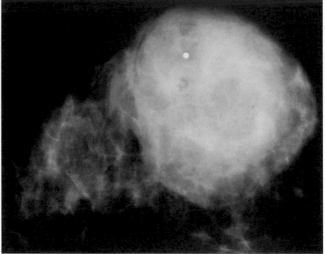

B

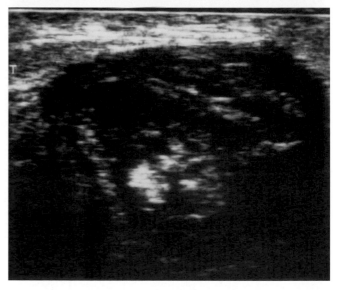

C

US-21. Invasive ductal carcinoma. The large, ill-defined mass on the MLO *(A)* and CC *(B)* projections in the subareolar right breast was complex on ultrasound *(C)*. It proved to be a large invasive carcinoma that contained cystic areas.

Teaching Point: The imaging appearance of this lesion is nonspecific. It is indistinguishable from an intracystic bleed or even an abscess.

FALSE-NEGATIVE ULTRASOUND

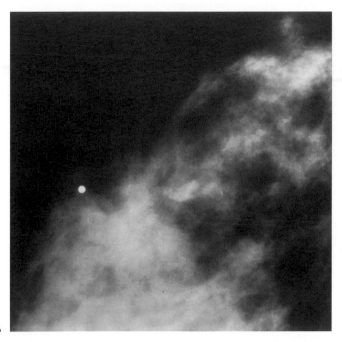

A

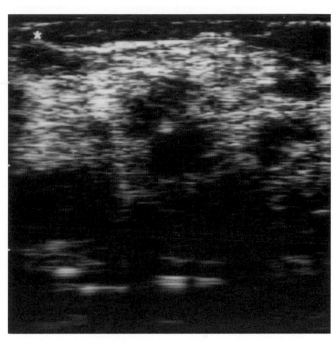

B

US-22. False-negative ultrasound. The palpable mass appears as an irregular, spiculated, 1.5-cm mass on spot compression mammography *(A)*. No focal mass was visible on the ultrasound *(B)*. There were scattered, hypoechoic areas throughout the area. At biopsy, a single, grade II, invasive ductal carcinoma was found.

Teaching Point: Breast cancer can be isoechoic with normal tissue.

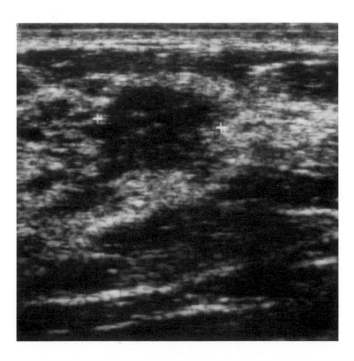

US-23. Occult cancer found by ultrasound alone. This irregularly shaped hypoechoic mass with isoechoic retrotumoral tissues and a heterogeneous echotexture was found by accident while what proved to be a fibroadenoma was being scanned. Even with the knowledge of its location, it was not visible on mammography.

Teaching Point: Although the data do not support ultrasound for screening apparently asymptomatic, mammographically negative tissues, cases such as this raise the question of whether or not ultrasound should be revisited as a possible second-level screening test. Prospective studies are needed.

FALSE-POSITIVE ULTRASOUND

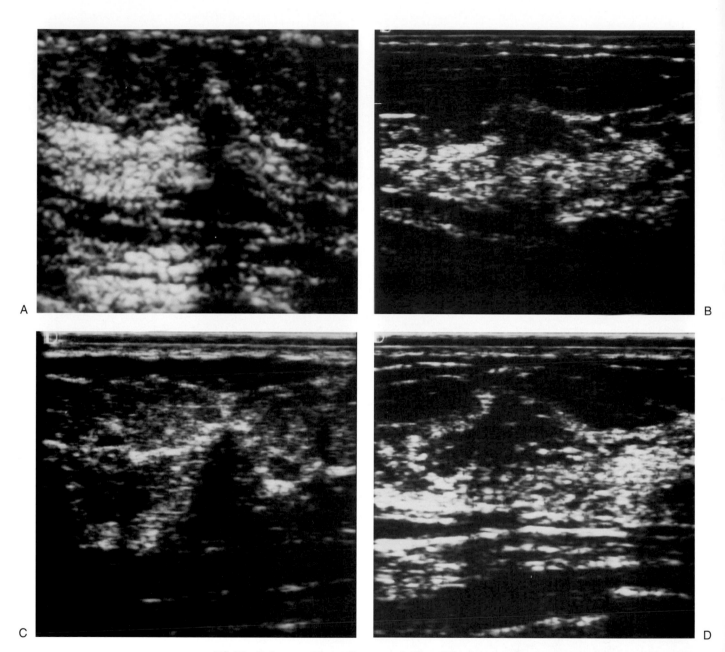

US-24. False-positive ultrasound. The difficulty of screening using ultrasound lies with the numerous "suspicious" areas that are found in virtually every woman. These four images *(A,B,C,D)* were all obtained in women with cysts by ultrasound. These images were in areas away from the cysts where there were no clinical or mammographic concerns. All of these hypoechoic areas could represent occult malignancies, but given the fact that they were obtained in women in their early 30s, with no other signs of breast cancer, they are unlikely to be small cancers, but rather normal tissue structures. Until criteria for intervention of lesions found only by ultrasound are defined, it is best to not survey breast tissue.

Teaching Point: Until screening using ultrasound is validated, and the parameters for intervention are defined, it is best to not go "looking around."

INVASIVE CARCINOMA

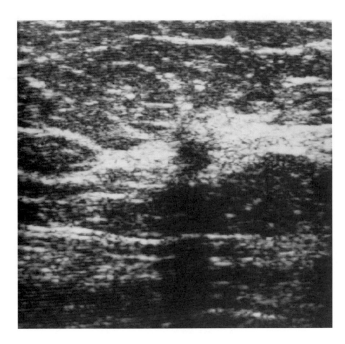

US-25. Small invasive breast cancer. This small (7 mm), irregularly shaped, hypoechoic mass with some posterior acoustic was first detected by mammography. This ultrasound was performed prior to ultrasound-guided core needle biopsy that revealed invasive breast cancer.

Teaching Point: Small cancers can be seen by ultrasound, but it is often difficult to find them because normal breast tissues can produce a similar appearance.

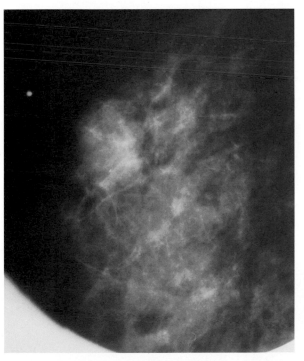

A

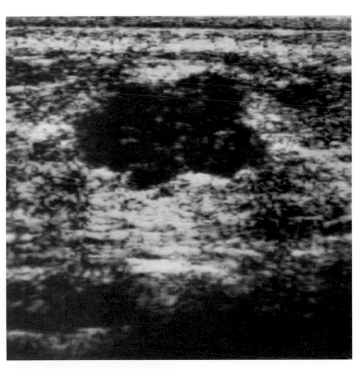

B

US-26. Invasive ductal carcinoma. A palpable mass developed in a 48-year-old woman. The spot compression magnification, tangential view *(A)*, showed the mass under the skin marker. It has a lobulated margin that is confirmed on the ultrasound study *(B)*, which reveals a well-defined but lobulated hypoechoic mass, enhanced through transmission of sound. Biopsy revealed invasive ductal carcinoma.

Teaching Point: Ultrasound is useful in the differentiation of cystic from solid masses. Breast cancer can have virtually any shape and echo characteristics on ultrasound.

LYMPH NODE EVALUATION

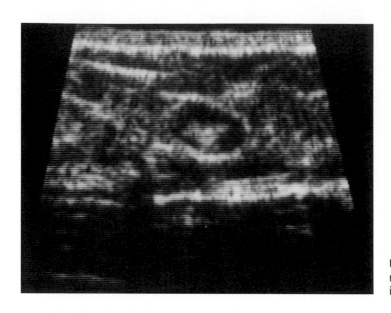

US-27. Intramammary lymph node. This hypoechoic mass with an echogenic center (pseudo-kidney) is benign intramammary lymph node as seen on ultrasound.

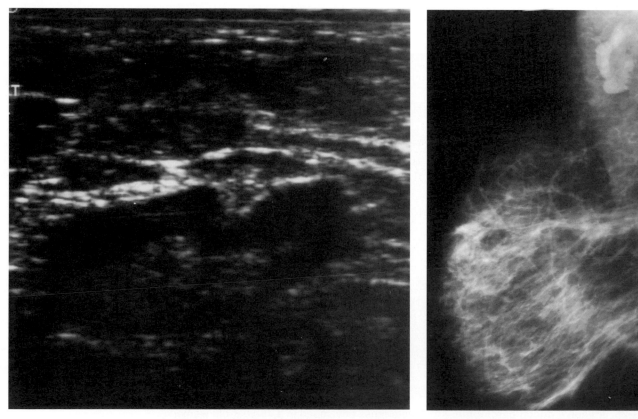

US-28. Axillary lymph node. A palpable area in the left axilla was evaluated with ultrasound, and its hypoechoic, lobulated appearance with an echogenic center *(A)* exactly mimics the large, fatty replaced lymph node seen on the mammogram *(B)*.

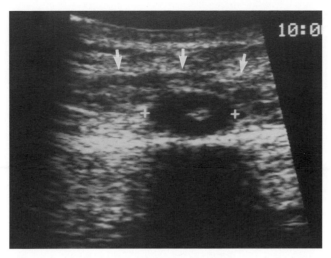

US-29. Pseudo-lymph node. Given that the pectoralis major *(arrows)* is anterior to this "mass" that is hypoechoic with an echogenic center (pseudo-kidney), this rib in cross section should not be mistaken for a mass or lymph node.

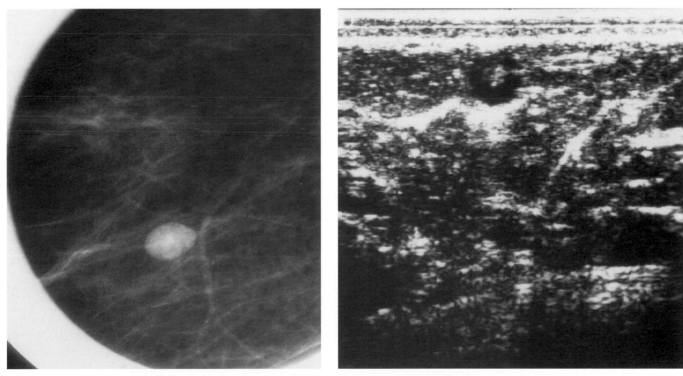

A   B

US-30. Pseudo-lymph node. This ovoid mass on mammography *(A)* was hypoechoic on ultrasound with an echogenic center *(B)*. It proved to be a simple cyst with thick fluid.

Teaching Point: All hypoechoic masses with echogenic centers are not lymph nodes.

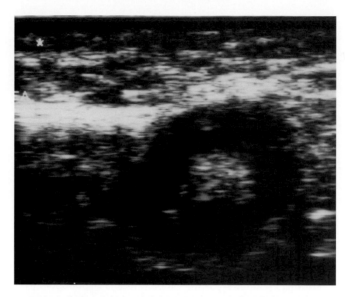

US-31. Metastatic breast cancer to an axillary lymph node. Despite the fact that there is echogenic tissue, suggestive of fat in the center of this hypoechoic lymph node, the node contained metastatic breast cancer.

Teaching Point: The appearance of fat, by ultrasound, in the center of a lymph node, does not ensure that the lymph node is normal.

Section VI:
Magnetic Resonance Imaging Atlas

Magnetic resonance imaging (MRI) is becoming increasingly useful in clinical breast evaluation. It represents the best method for imaging women with implants to discover possible rupture of the implant. It is an expensive but accurate way of differentiating cysts from solid masses. Gadolinium DTPA-enhanced imaging appears to be more accurate than mammography and clinical examination in predicting the extent of a cancer. More foci of breast cancer in the ipsilateral breast are found by MRI than by any other test. Although it may not be sufficiently accurate to avoid a safe breast biopsy, the rate of contrast enhancement and its pattern of washout can help to differentiate benign from malignant lesions. Although ductal carcinoma *in situ* may not always enhance, it appears to be extremely rare for an invasive breast cancer to not enhance following intravenous contrast administration.

Using gadolinium DTPA we have found a number of breast cancers in the contralateral breast of women being studied for ipsilateral lesions. These were totally unsuspected, and were not visible by mammography or ultrasound. This indicates that MRI may one day be useful for the detection of mammographically and clinically occult cancer of the breast. If the cost of doing MRI can be reduced, I believe that MRI will become an important second-level (after mammography and clinical breast examination) screening technique, particularly for women with dense or difficult to evaluate breast tissue. [See *Breast Imaging, Second Edition*, pp. 617–635]

ACKNOWLEDGMENTS

I am grateful to Priscilla Slanetz, M.D., Robert Weiskoff, Ph.D., and Whitney Edmister, who have done the breast MRI research in our group and have provided these cases.

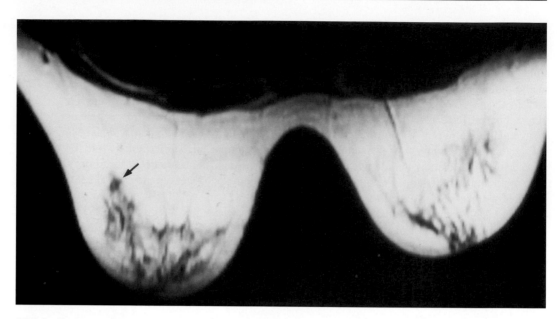

MR-1. Cancer without contrast enhancement. This small invasive ductal carcinoma is visible on this T1-weighted image *(arrow)* because it is surrounded by fat. However, its basic signal intensity is no different from the other fibroglandular structures, and it would not be visible if it had developed within normal fibroglandular structures.

Teaching Point: MRI without intravenous contrast enhancement has, thus far, not proven useful for cancer evaluation.

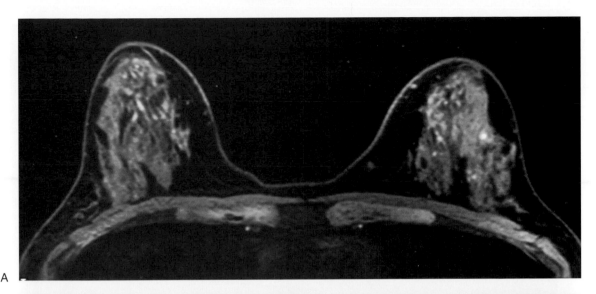

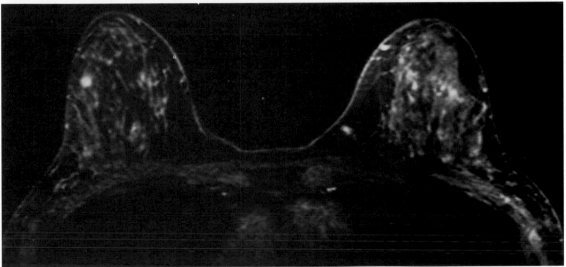

MR-2. Normal MRI. Using fat suppression techniques, the fat on these precontrast images is low in signal and the parenchymal tissues have a moderately high signal *(A)* on T1-weighted imaging using the gradient echo technique. Several minutes after the administration of gadolinium DTP, the parenchyma has increased in signal intensity with a patchy distribution *(B)*. Although there is a bright area in the lateral aspect of the right breast, no rapidly enhancing areas were identified and there is no evidence of malignancy on mammography or clinical breast examination.

Teaching Point: Although lesions surrounded by fat are easily seen by MRI without contrast enhancement, they are also easily visible by mammography at a much lower cost. Cancers developing in dense fibroglandular tissues are not easily seen by unenhanced breast MRI; consequently, unenhanced breast MRI did not prove useful for detecting or diagnosing breast cancer. Normal breast tissue and benign lesions can enhance, but the dynamics of the enhancement usually differ from that of cancer. Most invasive breast cancers demonstrate contrast enhancement following the intravenous administration of gadolinium and generally enhance more rapidly than normal tissues and benign lesions. Although the data remain inconclusive, a combination of morphologic characteristics and the dynamics of contrast enhancement will likely help in breast evaluation.

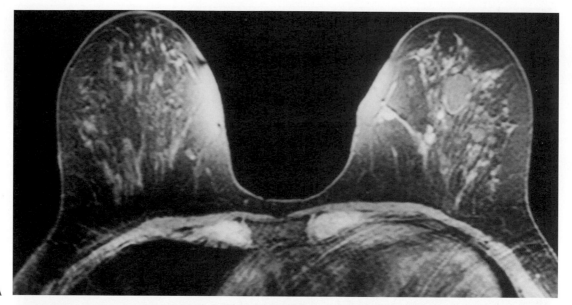

A

B

MR-3. Cysts. On T1-weighted imaging with fat suppression (TR 23, TE 6), the cyst in the left breast is low in signal intensity *(A)*. On T2-weighted imaging (TR 3,500, TE 102), the cyst becomes high in signal intensity *(B)*.

Teaching Point: Cysts produce a low signal intensity on T1-weighted images and a high signal intensity on T2-weighted images.

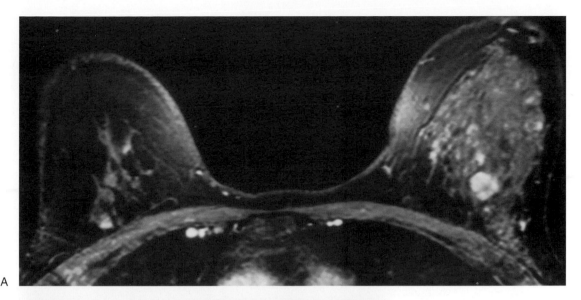

A

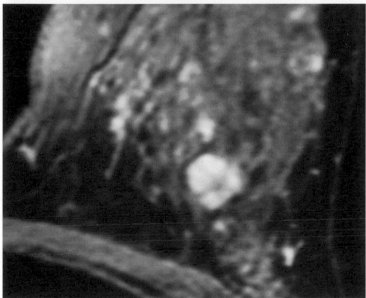

B

MR-4. Fibroadenoma. On T1-weighted imaging (TR 23, TE 6), the fibroadenoma in the left breast *(A)* has the typical lobulated appearance with low-signal-intensity septations [seen on the enlarged image *(B)*].

Teaching Point: Low-signal-intensity septations on T1-weighted images in a lobulated or ovoid mass with well-defined margins has a high diagnostic specificity for a benign fibroadenoma on MRI.

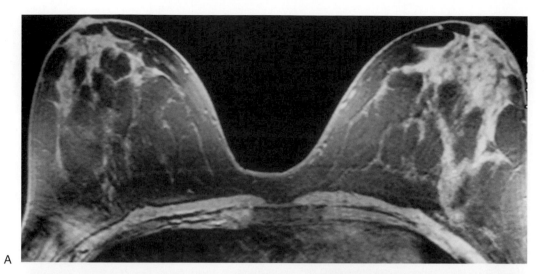

A

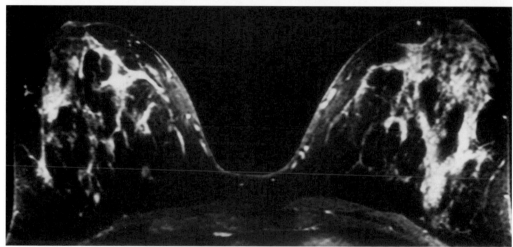

B

MR-5. Intraductal carcinoma (DCIS). Although there appears to be bilateral contrast enhancement when comparing the precontrast T1-weighted images (TR 23, TE 6) *(A)*, with the postcontrast T1-weighted images *(B)*, the dynamic imaging showed that the left breast tissues enhanced more rapidly than the right. The entire upper outer left breast down to the nipple was involved with high-grade DCIS.

Teaching Points: 1. The enhancement of DCIS may be variable or none at all when compared to the normal tissues. Furthermore, it is not merely the enhancement of tissues, since many normal tissues and benign lesions enhance, but the rate at which they enhance that helps to differentiate benign from malignant processes. The enhancement of DCIS is likely related to whether or not it has stimulated neovascularity, and this appears to vary between DCIS lesions. 2. Fat suppression is used to eliminate the bright signal from fat that can mask the signal enhancement of a lesion following gadolinium administration. If fat suppression is not available, and if pre- and postcontrast images can be accurately registered, the images can be subtracted to reveal areas of enhancement.

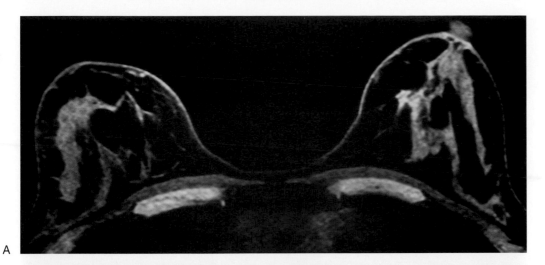

A

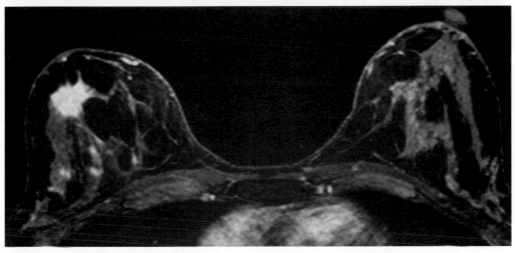

B

MR-6. Invasive ductal carcinoma. The palpable and mammographically visible cancer in the right breast was not visible on the precontrast T1-weighted image (TR 23, TE 6) *(A)*, but showed dramatic enhancement on the postcontrast study *(B)* also showing the classic irregular shape and spiculated margins of an invasive ductal carcinoma.

Teaching Point: Invasive ductal carcinomas virtually all enhance rapidly following the intravenous administration of contrast.

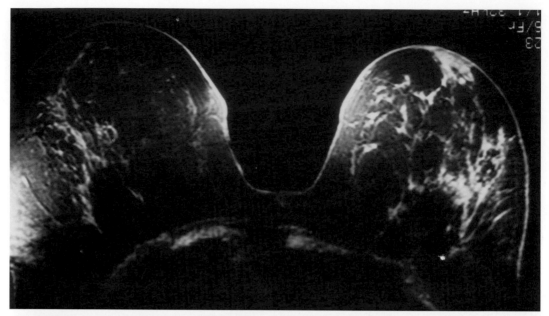

A

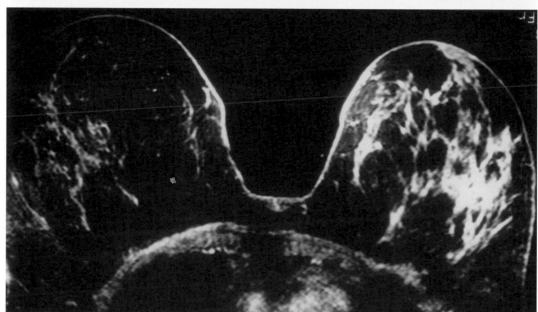

B

MR-7. Invasive lobular carcinoma. The asymmetric tissue on T1-weighted images (TR 23, TE 6) in the left breast *(A)* shows dramatic enhancement on postgadolinium imaging *(B)*.

Teaching Point: These cancers are notorious for developing insidiously. In our experience these cancers usually show dramatic enhancement, although several have shown little enhancement. MRI may be a method for their earlier detection.

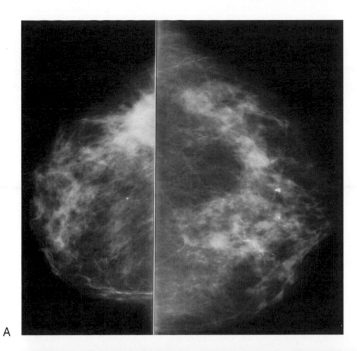

A

MR-8. Recurrent breast cancer. The recurrent breast cancer visible in the lateral aspect of the left breast on the CC projection and the new primary cancer in the medial right breast *(A)* enhance on the postgadolinium MRI. The recurrent breast cancer is much larger *(B)* than the new, contralateral primary cancer *(C).*

Teaching Point: MRI can be helpful in the detection of recurrent breast cancer. The easy visibility of the clinically occult contralateral cancer raises the hope that MRI may be useful as a second-level screening test.

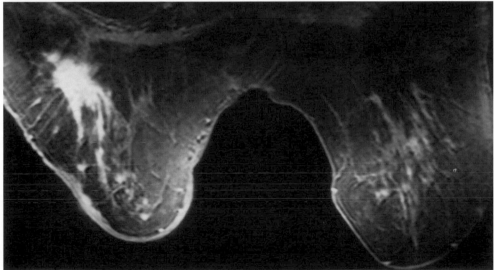

B

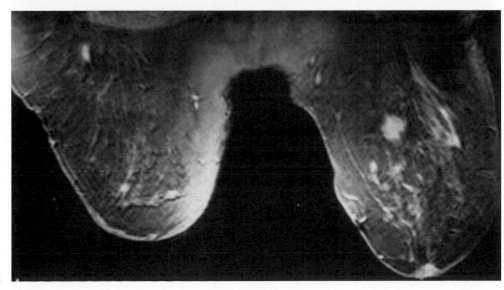

C

IMPLANT IMAGING

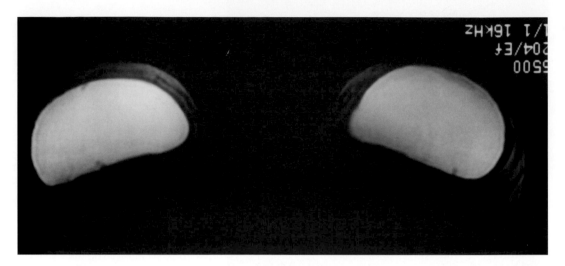

MR-9. MRI and normal silicone implants. Silicone is bright on T2-weighted imaging, as demonstrated in this study. Using fat and water suppression, only silicone gives a bright signal.

Teaching Point: Using fat and water suppression can help differentiate a fluid collection from silicone. Normal implants may have a lobulated or even irregular border. Rupture can never be excluded, but if silicone is seen outside the envelope, or the envelope is seen sinking into the gel, then rupture is almost certain.

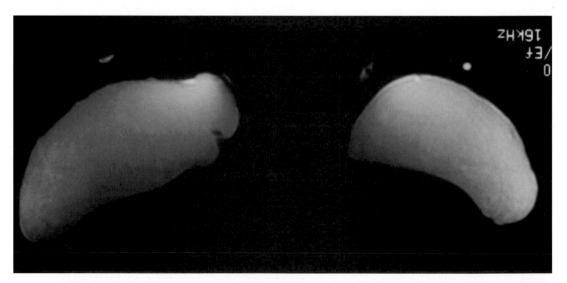

MR-10. Ruptured implant with free silicone. The implant on the right is ruptured as seen on this T2-weighted, fat-suppressed image, and free silicone gel is visible extravasating into the surrounding tissue medially. Its contour is somewhat preserved due to the cohesiveness of the silicone gel.

Teaching Point: MRI can demonstrate silicone outside an implant.

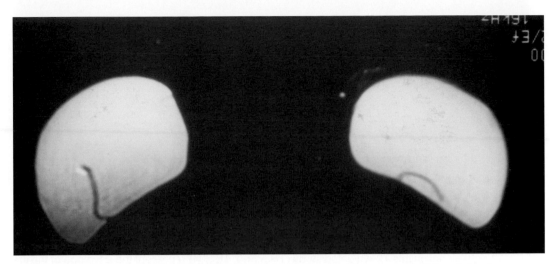

MR-11. Radial folds. The low signal intensity curvilinear structures on this T2-weighted, fat-suppressed image are merely invaginations of the intact silicone rubber envelope of the implants, which remain intact.

Teaching Point: When envelope material projects into the implant, but is continuous with the edge of the implant and there is no silicone between the folds ("teardrop" sign with silicone outside the envelope), then the structures represent infolding of the patulous envelope and do not represent a ruptured implant.

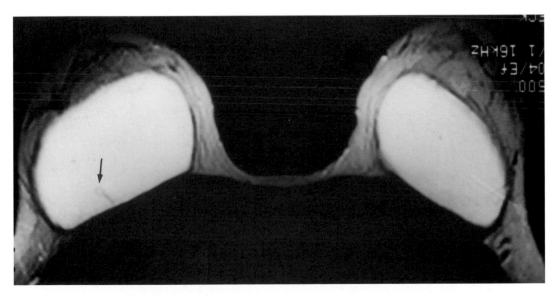

MR-12. Ruptured implant indicated by the "teardrop" sign. The low signal intensity structure at the back of the right implant looks like a "radial fold" on this water-suppressed image, but note that there is silicone in the loop of the fold, making the fold look like a teardrop (silicone on the inside and outside of the loop). The silicone inside the loop are outside the envelope of the implant, indicating that it has ruptured.

Teaching Point: The "teardrop" sign is the most subtle sign of an implant rupture. A "teardrop" must be differentiated from a radial fold, where volume averaging may make it appear that there is silicone in the loop. In the latter situation, the implants have not ruptured.

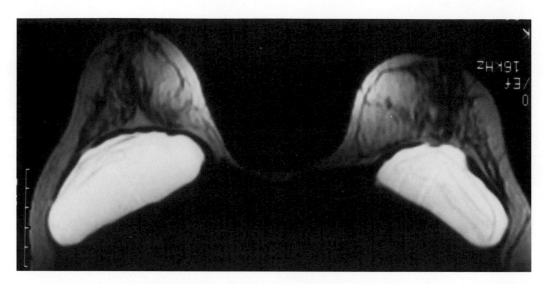

MR-13. Ruptured implants. The dark lines of low signal intensity that appear within the bright signal on this T2-weighted study (TR 5,500, TE 204) represent the envelope of the implant sinking into the silicone gel of these ruptured implants. The silicone remains contained within the fibrous capsule that had formed around the implants before the envelope ruptured.

Teaching Point: The "linguine" sign or the "fallen envelope" sign represents the ruptured implant sinking into the silicone gel. This represents the most accurate evidence of an implant rupture.

Subject Index

Page numbers followed by *f* refer to figures.